CAN: Camberwell Asses   d

A comprehensive needs assessment tool for people with severe mental illness

Mike Slade
Graham Thornicroft
Linda Loftus
Michael Phelan
Til Wykes

Published by Gaskell
London

Gaskell is an imprint of the Royal College of Psychiatrists,
17 Belgrave Square, London SW1X 8PG

Gaskell is a registered trademark of the Royal College of Psychiatrists.

British Library Cataloguing-in-Publication Data
A catalogue record for this book is available from the British Library.

ISBN 1-901242-25-0

Distributed in North America
by American Psychiatric Press, Inc.
ISBN 0-88048-595-7

The views presented in this book do not necessarily reflect those of the Royal College of Psychiatrists, and the publishers are not responsible for any error of omission or fact.

The Royal College of Psychiatrists is a registered charity (no. 228636)

Printed by Henry Ling Ltd., Dorchester, Dorset

Contents

Acknowledgements

Many people have contributed to the work reported in this book. The CAN was developed by a group which also included Graham Dunn, Frank Holloway and Geraldine Strathdee. Paul McCrone was an author of the first CAN paper, and currently coordinates translations. Subsequent papers have used data collected as part of the PRiSM Psychosis Study, and all the interviewers for this study are thanked, in particular Sue Parkman. The statistical contribution of Morven Leese has been invaluable. Other people who have contributed to the development and dissemination of the CAN include Thomas Becker, Liz Brooks, Sonia Johnson, George Szmukler and Ruth Taylor.

List of abbreviations

CAN   Camberwell Assessment of Need, a family of assessment schedules, currently including CANSAS, CAN–C and CAN–R
CANSAS   Camberwell Assessment of Need Short Appraisal Schedule
CAN–C   Camberwell Assessment of Need – Clinical version
CAN–R   Camberwell Assessment of Need – Research version
MRC   Medical Research Council
PRiSM   The Psychiatric Research in Service Measurement team is the Section of Community Psychiatry at the Institute of Psychiatry
SMI   Severely mentally ill

1 Introduction

The Camberwell Assessment of Need (CAN) is a tool for assessing the needs of people with severe and enduring mental illness. It covers a wide range of health and social needs, and incorporates both staff and user[1] assessment. The CAN was developed for use by:

(a) professionals who are involved in the care of people with severe mental illness;
(b) people wanting to evaluate mental health services; or
(c) service users in rating their own needs.

It was developed by the Section of Community Psychiatry (PRiSM), Institute of Psychiatry, Denmark Hill, London SE5 8AF, England.

This book is intended for people who are currently using or considering using the CAN. It provides a brief introduction to the subject of needs assessment in mental health, a comprehensive account of the development of the CAN, a manual for using three versions of the CAN, a training package, and answers to some frequently asked questions. Also included are copies (for photocopying) of the research, clinical and short versions of the CAN. Each chapter in this book is intended to be self-contained, which results in intentional duplication within Chapters 4–6.

The decision as to which parts of the book are relevant is made on the basis of the purpose of the needs assessment.

"I want to start using a needs assessment questionnaire in my clinical practice."
Read Chapter 2 for background, then look at CANSAS (Appendix 1) and CAN–C (Appendix 2). Decide whether the extra information assessed in CAN–C is needed, and then read Chapter 4 for CANSAS or Chapter 5 for CAN–C. If a team is going to start using the CAN, run a training session based on Chapter 7.

"I want to use a needs assessment schedule as an outcome measure in a research study."
Read Chapters 2 and 3 for background, then look at CANSAS (Appendix 1) and CAN–R (Appendix 4). Decide whether the extra information assessed in CAN–R is needed, and then read Chapter 4 for CANSAS or Chapter 6 for CAN–R. Use Chapter 7 when training interviewers.

"I've got a specific question about the CAN."
Read Chapter 8 for the answers to some frequently asked questions.

---

1. The term 'user' is used to indicate a person who is the subject of assessment using the CAN. This generic term is employed because the CAN is intended for use in both health and social services settings.

2 Needs assessment

A consistent theme to emerge from evolving community mental health care services during the past decade has been the recognition of the importance of a needs-led approach towards the individual care of those with severe mental illness (SMI). In the UK, this is a central theme in mental health policy (National Health Service and Community Care Act 1990), encouraged by the introduction of the Care Programme Approach. However, despite the wide recognition that people with SMI usually have a wide range of clinical and social needs, there is continuing confusion and debate about how such needs should be defined and assessed (Holloway, 1993).

The concept of need

There are a variety of approaches to defining need. The American psychologist Maslow established a hierarchy of need when attempting to formulate a theory of human motivation (Maslow, 1954). His belief was that fundamental physiological needs, such as the need for food, underpinned the higher needs of safety, love, self-esteem and self-actualisation. He proposed that people are motivated by the requirement to meet these needs, and that higher needs could only be met once the lower and more fundamental needs were met. This approach can be illustrated by the example of a homeless man, who is not concerned about his lack of friends while he is cold and hungry. However, once these needs have been met he may express more interest in having the company of other people.

Since the work of Maslow, other approaches have been developed for defining need with respect to health care. In the MRC Needs for Care Assessment, a need is defined as being present when a person's level of functioning falls below, or threatens to fall below, some specified level, and when there is some remediable, or potentially remediable, cause (Brewin *et al*, 1987). The sociologist Bradshaw (1972) proposed a taxonomy of three types of need: that which is either 'felt' or 'expressed' by the user; 'normative' need which is assessed by an expert; and 'comparative' need which arises from comparison with other groups or individuals. Such an approach helps to emphasise that need is a subjective concept, and that the judgement of whether a need is present or not will, in part, depend on whose viewpoint is being taken. Slade (1994) has discussed this issue with respect to differences in perception between the users of mental health services and the involved professionals, and he has argued that once differences are identified, then negotiation between staff and user can take place to agree a care plan.

Stevens & Gabbay (1991) have distinguished need (the ability to benefit in some way from health care), demand (wish expressed by the service user) and supply of services. These concepts can be illustrated by different components of mental health services. For instance, mental health services for homeless mentally ill people are rarely demanded by homeless people, but most professionals would agree that a need exists. In contrast, the demand for counselling services frequently outstrips supply.

Clearly, the need, demand and supply of services will never be perfectly matched. If mismatch is to be minimised then two fundamental principles must underpin mental health service development. First, services must try to address the identified problems and difficulties of local users (i.e. local services should be shaped by the specific needs of the population rather than being provided in line with any national template or historical patterns). Second, a continued effort to demonstrate what is, and is not, effective with different groups is required, so that resources are provided for effective interventions and not driven by demand or short-term political pressures.

Assessment of population need

If mental health services are to be developed in response to the needs of specific populations, and resources allocated on the basis of identified need, agreed methods for assessing population need for mental health services are required. The ideal method is to identify all individuals with mental health needs, and aggregate the results of their individual need assessments. Such an approach is rarely feasible, and in its place a range of proxy measures have been developed to estimate the need for mental health services within given populations. Current service utilisation rates are an inadequate measure of local need, as they are largely dependent on current provision. This is especially true in services which are already over-prescribed, such as inner-city in-patient beds. Measures of social deprivation which predict the prevalence of SMI and service utilisation (Jarman, 1983; Thornicroft, 1991) can be used to allocate resources. The Mental Illness Needs Index (Glover et al, 1998) uses census data to give an approximate estimate of local need. Although such approaches can help to guide the allocation of resources, it is vital that specific local factors are also taken into consideration, such as the presence of a large psychiatric hospital, which may have resulted in many ex-patients being settled in the surrounding area. Another approach is to compare local provision with national figures, which gives a crude comparison.

Individual needs assessment instruments

There is no perfect individual needs assessment tool. The requirements of different users vary, and there is inevitable conflict between factors such as brevity and comprehensiveness. Johnson et al (1996) summarised the features of an ideal needs assessment for use in clinical settings as brief, easily learned, quickly administered by clinical staff, valid and reliable. Numerous instruments have been developed by individual teams around the country to aid care planning and reviews. There is little consistency in the information that is collected, with a tendency to concentrate on qualitative, rather than quantitative, data. Psychometric properties are frequently ignored. Although the development of such instruments helps to focus a team's approach, they do not provide valid or accurate information to service planners.

One established needs assessment tool is the CAN (Phelan et al, 1995), which is the focus of this book. Other carefully designed needs assessment instruments include:

MRC Needs for Care Assessment

The MRC Needs for Care Assessment (Brewin et al, 1987) was designed to identify areas of remediable need. Need is defined as being present when a patient's functioning (social disablement) falls below, or threatens to fall below, some minimum specified level, and this is due to a remediable, or potentially remediable, cause. A need is defined as being met when it has attracted an item of care which is at least partly effective, and when no other item of care of greater potential effectiveness exists. A need is said to be unmet when it has only attracted a partly effective or no item of care, and when other items of care of greater potential effectiveness exist. The MRC Needs for Care Assessment has proved itself to be a robust research instrument, and there is a substantial body of research describing its use (Brewin et al, 1988; LeSage et al, 1991; Van Haaster et al, 1994; O'Leary & Webb, 1996). However, it is probably too complex and time consuming for routine clinical use, and difficulties have arisen when it has been used among long-term in-patients (Pryce et al, 1993) and the homeless mentally ill (Hogg & Marshall, 1992).

Cardinal Needs Schedule

The Cardinal Needs Schedule (Marshall, 1994) is a modification of the MRC Needs for Care Assessment. It identifies cardinal problems which satisfy three criteria:

(a) the "cooperation criterion" (the patient is willing to accept help for the problem);

(b) the "co-stress criterion" (the problem causes considerable anxiety, frustration or inconvenience to people caring for the patient); and

(c) the "severity criterion" (the problem endangers the health or safety of the patient, or the safety of other people).

The instrument involves a mental state assessment, the REHAB behaviour rating scale (Baker & Hall, 1988) and a specially designed additional information questionnaire. A computerised version known as AUTONEED is also available. Again, given the detail of this instrument, it is probably more suited to experienced researchers.

Bangor Assessment of Need Profile

The Bangor Assessment of Need Profile (Carter et al, 1996) comprises a self-report schedule designed to give a brief and simple indication of the expressed need of people with a long-term mental illness, and a schedule to assess need as perceived by a key informant. Need is present when an item falls below that which the respondent (user or key informant) perceives to be normal or ordinary functioning, and absent when the respondent perceives normal and independent functioning. Reliability is explored, and the instrument is primarily intended for research use.

3 Development of the Camberwell Assessment of Need (CAN)

Four broad principles governed the development of the CAN. First, that everyone has needs, and that although people with SMI have some specific needs, the majority of their needs are similar to those of people who do not have a mental illness, such as having somewhere to live, something to do and enough money. Second, it was clear that the majority of people with SMI have multiple needs, and that it is vital that all of them are identified by those caring for them. Therefore a priority of the CAN is to identify, rather than describe in detail, serious needs. Specialist assessments can be conducted in specific areas if required, once the need is identified. Third, needs assessment should be both an integral part of routine clinical practice and a component of service evaluation, so the CAN should be useable by a wide range of staff. Lastly, the CAN is based on the principle that need is a subjective concept, and that there will frequently be differing but equally valid perceptions about the presence or absence of a specific need. The CAN therefore records the views of staff and users separately.

The specific criteria that were established for the CAN are that it:

(a)   has adequate psychometric properties;
(b)   can be completed within 30 minutes;
(c)   can be used by a wide range of professionals;
(d)   is suitable for both routine clinical practice and research;
(e)   can be learnt and used, without formal training;
(f)   incorporates the views of both users and staff about needs;
(g)   measures both met and unmet need; and
(h)   measures the level of help received from friends or relatives as well as from statutory services.

Psychometric properties

The reliability and validity of the CAN have been described in detail elsewhere (Phelan *et al*, 1995) (see Appendix 7). In brief, the selection of items to be included in the CAN was guided by validity studies, including surveys of people with SMI and mental health professionals. In a study of people with SMI attending an inner-city mental health service, the mean number of needs identified by staff was 7.55 and by patients 8.64. Correlations of the inter-rater and test–retest reliability of the total number of needs identified by staff were 0.99 and 0.78, respectively. The percentage complete agreement on individual items ranged from 81.6 to 100% (inter-rater) and 58.1 to 100% (test–retest).

The CAN has been developed incrementally, and CAN 3.0 is now in use (and discussed in this book). The original version was developed for research use, and called CAN–R. Two variants have also been developed: a short clinical version (CANSAS) and a long clinical version (CAN–C). All versions assess need in the same 22 domains, and can be used to assess the views of both users and staff. Chapters 4–6 provide details on using each of these CAN variants.

4 Using the Camberwell Assessment of Need Short Appraisal Schedule (CANSAS)

The Camberwell Assessment of Need Short Appraisal (CANSAS) is a short (single page) summary of the needs of a mental health service user. The CANSAS can be used in clinical settings because it is short enough to be used for review purposes on a routine basis. It can also be used as an outcome measure in research studies, especially when a number of assessment schedules are being used. A copy of the CANSAS is shown in Appendix 1, and may be photocopied freely for your use.

The CANSAS assesses 22 domains of health and social needs:

1 Accommodation
2 Food
3 Looking after the home
4 Self-care
5 Daytime activities
6 Physical health
7 Psychotic symptoms
8 Information on condition and treatment
9 Psychological distress
10 Safety to self
11 Safety to others
12 Alcohol
13 Drugs
14 Company
15 Intimate relationships
16 Sexual expression
17 Child care
18 Basic education
19 Telephone
20 Transport
21 Money
22 Benefits

Questions are asked about each domain, to identify (a) whether a need or problem is present in that domain; and (b) whether the need is met or unmet. A need is met if there is currently not a problem in the domain, but a problem would exist if it were not for the help provided (i.e. they are getting effective help). A need is unmet if there is currently a problem in the domain (whether or not any help is currently being provided). At the end of an assessment, therefore, it will be possible to say how many needs the user has from these 22 domains, and how many of these needs are unmet.

Note A CANSAS assessment by itself is wide-ranging ('comprehensive'), but not thorough, because a person can have needs in a particular domain for a variety of reasons. The CANSAS is therefore not an adequate assessment on which to decide whether to offer help, but should be used to identify domains in which more assessment is needed.

Each CANSAS sheet can be used to make up to four assessments. One use would be to record staff and user assessments of need before and after an intervention. Another use would be to record the perceptions of a range of people at a specific point in time, such as the user, informal care-giver, keyworker and general practitioner. A third use would be to review changes in needs over time.

An assessment using the CANSAS involves an interviewer asking an interviewee questions about each of the 22 domains. The interviewer should be a professional with some knowledge of the difficulties which can be involved in interviewing people with SMI, such as impaired concentration, disorganisation and psychotic symptoms. The interviewer should also be familiar with issues relating to safety and confidentiality, as discussed by Parkman & Bixby (1996).

Administration of the CANSAS

Each CANSAS assessment is recorded in a separate column. Thus one CANSAS sheet can be used for up to four assessments. The interviewee may be the user, the carer (e.g. a friend or family member) or a member of staff (e.g. the keyworker). If the user or carer is being interviewed, administration involves the interviewer going through the CANSAS, asking the user about each domain in turn. If a member of staff is the interviewee, this normally involves the member of staff filling in the CANSAS.

Whoever is being interviewed, it is important that it is their views which are assessed. Specifically, there are no 'right' or 'wrong' answers. So, for example, the staff members should give their own views about the user's needs, rather than what they think the user's views are.

Before starting the assessment, the date of assessment and the assessor's initials are recorded in the box at the top of the column. An interview with the user is indicated by circling 'U' at the top of the relevant column, with the carer by circling 'C', and with the staff by circling 'S'. Each of the 22 domains is then assessed, in the order shown (see Appendix 1).

Note Anchor points and some of the opening questions which appear in the CAN–C and CAN–R have been omitted from the CANSAS. It is therefore recommended that interviewers familiarise themselves with the full Section 1 for each domain (shown in CAN–R and CAN–C). This could be done by completing Section 1 from CAN–R or CAN–C for the first few assessments, and transcribing the results onto the CANSAS form.

The purpose of the interview should be explained. For the user, this explanation might take the form "I'd like to go through this questionnaire with you, which covers a whole range of areas of life in which people can have difficulties. I'll go through each of these areas in turn, and ask about any problems you have had in the last month. Is that okay?".

Time should be allowed for questions, and to ensure that the assessment is not rushed. A typical CANSAS assessment should take five minutes, but this will be affected by the number of needs identified and characteristics of the interviewee. For example, if the user has difficulties with concentration, then a break may be needed during the interview.

Assessment of each domain is identical. A suggested opening question is shown on the CANSAS in italics, and where necessary follow-up questions should be asked, with the goal of establishing (a) whether the user experiences any problems in this domain; and (b) if they do experience problems, whether they are getting effective help. On the basis of the interviewee's responses, a need rating is made:

0 = no serious problem   (no need)
1 = no/moderate problem due to help given   (met need)
2 = serious problem   (unmet need)
9 = not known

The need rating is made using the following algorithm:

If the interviewee does not know or does not want to answer questions on this domain then rate **9** (not known)

otherwise

If a serious problem is present (regardless of cause, or whether any help is being given or not) then rate **2** (unmet need)

otherwise

If there is no serious problem because of help given then rate **1** (met need)

otherwise

Rate **0** (no need)

Note   Just because there is currently no problem, the need rating is not automatically 0. For example, a person with diabetes who is physically well because of the prescribed insulin would be rated as 1 (met need) for physical health.

Note   A need can exist for a variety of reasons. For example, a person with a psychotic illness may currently be unable to do his or her shopping because of a sprained ankle. He or she should be rated as having a need (i.e. need rating 1 or 2) in the Food domain, even though this need is not related to his or her psychiatric condition.

For each domain, anchor points for the need ratings can be referred to in CAN–R and CAN–C. However, the difference between rating 1 and 2 can be a matter of judgement. The goal is to differentiate between problems which are current and severe and those which are ameliorated by help, but there may still be a blurred boundary where the user is receiving help which only partly addresses his or her difficulties. Be guided by the interviewee's response – does he or she see the problem as current and severe (need rating 2), or under control with the help that the user is getting (need rating 1)?

For some of the 22 domains, there are some specific issues which have been found to require clarification.

1   Accommodation

If a person is currently in hospital and does not have a home to be discharged to, the need rating should be 1. If a person is currently in hospital and does have an appropriate home to be discharged to, the need rating should be 0 (this is an example of overmet need, which the CANSAS does not assess).

2   Food

A need is present if the person is not getting an adequate diet, due to difficulties with shopping, storage and/or cooking of food, or because inadequate or culturally inappropriate food is being provided (e.g. by a hospital ward). However, if the problem is primarily due to difficulties with budgeting then this should be rated under the domain of Money, and the Food rating should be 0.

3   Looking after the home

This domain concerns difficulties in maintaining the living environment, whether this is a hostel room or an independent home. It may not be possible for staff to rate this if the person is homeless, but the user may be able to state whether he or she believes that it would be a problem if he or she had a home.

4   Self-care

This domain refers to personal hygiene, and does not include untidiness or bizarre appearance.

5   Daytime activities

If the user is unable to occupy him- or herself during the day without help then he or she has a need in this domain. Help given might include sheltered employment, attending a day centre, or activities with friends and relatives. If the primary problem is loneliness rather than boredom then this should be rated under the domain of Company.

6   Physical health

Physical side-effects of medication should be considered, as well as any acute or chronic medical or dental condition.

7   Psychotic symptoms

When asking the user about this domain particular care should be taken to record his or her perceptions. For example, a user who denies hearing voices and having problems with his or her thoughts, and states that the depot injection is to keep him or her calm, should be rated as 0 (no need).

8   Information on condition and treatment

This should include information about local service provision, as well as information about the user's specific condition.

9   Psychological distress

This should include depression and anxiety, regardless of the cause.

10   Safety to self

Risk due to severe self-neglect or vulnerability to exploitation should also be rated, as well as risk of suicide and self-harm.

11   Safety to others

Inadvertent risks (e.g. fire risk due to careless use of cigarettes) should be included, as well as risk of deliberate violence.

16   Sexual expression

This includes difficulties due to medication side-effects, as well as a lack of safe sex practices and inadequate contraception.

20   Transport

A need should be rated if a person is unable to use public transport for physical or psychological reasons.

21   Money

This refers to ability to cope with the available amount of money. If the user says that he or she does not have enough money, this should be assessed in the domain of Benefits.

At the end of the assessment, add up the number of met needs (need rating 1), and record in row A. Add up the number of unmet needs (need rating 2), and record in row B. Add these two number to give the total number of domains in which a need has been assessed, and record this figure in row C.

Using information from a CANSAS assessment

How CANSAS assessment information is used will depend on why the assessment is being made. Information can be used for at least three purposes:

(a)   CANSAS data can be used at the level of the individual user, by providing a baseline measure of level of need, or for charting changes in the user over time. For example, one approach would be to use the CANSAS routinely in initial assessments of new service users, to identify the range of domains in which they are likely to require further assessment and (possibly) help or treatment.

(b)   CANSAS data can be used for auditing and developing an individual service. For example, to investigate:

(i)   the impact on needs of providing an intervention for a group of service users, by looking at changes across this group;

(ii)   case load dependency for different workers;

(iii)   whether enough users have unmet needs in the domain of Benefits to make it worthwhile for a community mental health team to employ a welfare benefits advisor.

(c)   The CANSAS can be used as an outcome measure for research purposes, such as the impact on needs of two different types of mental health services, or the reasons why staff and service user perceptions differ.

5 Using the Camberwell Assessment of Need – Clinical version (CAN–C)

The Camberwell Assessment of Need – Clinical version (CAN–C) is intended for clinical use, and is shown in Appendix 2, with summary score sheets in Appendix 3. It may be photocopied freely for your use.

The CAN–C has four sections for each domain, and is completed separately by the staff and service user. Section 1 assesses the need rating (no need, met need, unmet need or not known) for the domain. The purpose of Section 1 is twofold. First, to assess whether there is a need in the domain, and whether effective help is already being given. Second, to decide whether further questions about this domain are necessary. Section 2 assesses the amount of help from informal sources (friends, relatives, etc.). Section 3 assesses the amount of help given by and needed from formal services. For all ratings, anchor points and rating guidelines are provided. Section 4 records the user's perceptions about the domain, and the staff care plan.

The CAN–C assesses 22 domains of health and social needs.

1   Accommodation
2   Food
3   Looking after the home
4   Self-care
5   Daytime activities
6   Physical health
7   Psychotic symptoms
8   Information on condition and treatment
9   Psychological distress
10 Safety to self
11 Safety to others
12 Alcohol
13 Drugs
14 Company
15 Intimate relationships
16 Sexual expression
17 Child care
18 Basic education
19 Telephone
20 Transport
21 Money
22 Benefits

Questions are asked about each domain, to identify:

(a) Whether a need or problem is present in that domain. A need is met if there is currently not a problem in the domain, but a problem would exist if it were not for the help provided (i.e. they are getting effective help). A need is unmet if there is currently a problem in the domain (whether or not any help is currently being provided).

(b) Whether the need is met or unmet.

(c) How much help the user is currently receiving from informal (friends, family, etc.) or formal sources, and how much help he or she needs.

(d) The user's views about his or her needs.

Space is also provided for staff to record the care plan relevant to this domain.

At the end of an assessment, therefore, it will be possible to say how many needs the user has from these 22 domains, what help he or she is currently receiving and what help is needed, and what his or her perspective is about the difficulties.

Note A CAN–C assessment by itself may not be sufficient, so the care plan may identify a need for further assessment.

Each CAN–C can be used to record the perceptions of the staff and the user. To avoid bulky notes, one-page summary sheets are provided in Appendix 3, which are suitable for case notes.

An assessment using CAN–C involves an interviewer asking an interviewee questions about each of 22 domains. The interviewer should be a professional with some knowledge of the difficulties which can be involved in interviewing people with SMI, such as impaired concentration, disorganisation and psychotic symptoms. The interviewer should also be familiar with issues relating to safety and confidentiality, as discussed by Parkman & Bixby (1996).

Administration of the CAN–C

The interviewee may be the user or a member of staff (e.g. the keyworker). If the user is being interviewed, administration involves the interviewer going through the CAN–C, asking the user about each domain in turn. If a member of staff is the interviewee, this normally involves the member of staff filling in the CAN–C.

Whoever is being interviewed, it is important that it is their views which are assessed. Specifically, there are no 'right' or 'wrong' answers. So, for example, the staff members should give their own views about the users' needs, rather than what they think the users' views are.

The purpose of the interview should be explained to the user. This explanation might take the form, "I'd like to go through this questionnaire with you, which covers a whole range of areas of life in which people can have difficulties. I'll go through each of these areas in turn, and ask about any problems you have had in the last month. Is that okay?". Time should be allowed for questions, and to ensure that the assessment is not rushed. A typical CAN–C assessment should take 15–20 minutes, but this will be affected by the number of needs identified and characteristics of the interviewee. For example, if the user has difficulties with concentration, then a break may be needed during the interview.

Each of the 22 domains is assessed, in the order shown. Each domain comprises four sections. For each domain, care should be taken to ensure that the correct column (staff or user) is completed.

Section 1

Suggested opening questions are given in italics for each domain. Where necessary, follow-up questions can be asked, with the goal of establishing (a) whether the user experiences any problems in this

14

domain; and (b) if the user does experience problems, is he or she getting effective help. On the basis of the interviewee's responses, a need rating is made:

0 = no serious problem   (no need)
1 = no/moderate problem due to help given   (met need)
2 = serious problem   (unmet need)
9 = not known

The need rating is made using the following algorithm:

If the interviewee does not know or does not want to answer questions on this domain then rate **9** (not known)

otherwise

If a serious problem is present (regardless of cause, or whether any help is being given or not) then rate **2** (unmet need)

otherwise

If there is no serious problem because of help given then rate **1** (met need)

otherwise

Rate **0** (no need)

Note Just because there is currently no problem, the need rating is not automatically 0. For example, a person with diabetes who is physically well because of the prescribed insulin would be rated as 1 (met need) for physical health.

Note A need can exist for a variety of reasons. For example, a person with a psychotic illness may currently be unable to do his or her shopping because of a sprained ankle. He or she should be rated as having a need (i.e. need rating 1 or 2) in the Food domain, even though this need is not related to his or her psychiatric condition.

For each domain, anchor points for the need ratings can be referred to in CAN–C. However, the difference between rating 1 and 2 can be a matter of judgement. The goal is to differentiate between problems which are current and severe and those which are ameliorated by help, but there may still be a blurred boundary where the user is receiving help which only partly addresses his or her difficulties. Be guided by the interviewee's response – does he or she they see the problem as current and severe (need rating 2), or under control with the help that the user is getting (need rating 1)?

For some of the 22 domains, there are some specific issues in Section 1 which have been found to require clarification.

1   Accommodation

If a person is currently in hospital and does not have a home to be discharged to, the need rating should be 1. If a person is currently in hospital and does have an appropriate home to be discharged to, the need rating should be 0 (this is an example of overmet need, which the CAN–C does not assess).

2   Food

A need is present if the person is not getting an adequate diet, due to difficulties with shopping, storage and/or cooking of food, or because inadequate or culturally inappropriate food is being provided (e.g. by a hospital ward). However, if the problem is primarily due to difficulties with budgeting then this should be rated under the domain of Money, and the Food rating should be 0.

3   Looking after the home

This domain concerns difficulties in maintaining the living environment, whether this is a hostel room or an independent home. It may not be possible for staff to rate this if the person is homeless, but the user may be able to state whether he or she believes that it would be a problem if he or she had a home.

4   Self-care

This domain refers to personal hygiene, and does not include untidiness or bizarre appearance.

5   Daytime activities

If the user is unable to occupy him- or herself during the day without help, then he or she has a need in this domain. Help given might include sheltered employment, attending a day centre, or activities with friends and relatives. If the primary problem is loneliness rather than boredom then this should be rated under the domain of Company.

6   Physical health

Physical side-effects of medication should be considered, as well as any acute or chronic medical or dental condition.

7   Psychotic symptoms

When asking the user about this domain particular care should be taken to record his or her perceptions. For example, a user who denies hearing voices and having problems with thoughts, and states that the depot injection is to keep him or her calm, should be rated as 0 (no need).

8   Information

This should include information about local service provision, as well as information about the user's specific condition.

9   Psychological distress

This should include depression and anxiety, regardless of the cause.

10   Safety to self

Risk due to severe self-neglect or vulnerability to exploitation should also be rated, as well as risk of suicide and self-harm.

11   Safety to others

Inadvertent risks (e.g. fire risk due to careless use of cigarettes) should be included, as well as risk of deliberate violence.

16   Sexual expression

This includes difficulties due to medication side-effects, as well as a lack of safe sex practices and inadequate contraception.

20   Transport

A need should be rated if a person is unable to use public transport for physical or psychological reasons.

21   Money

This refers to ability to cope with the available amount of money. If the user says that he or she does not have enough money, this should be assessed in the domain of Benefits.

If the rating is 0 or 9 go on to the next domain on the following page. If the rating is 1 or 2 (i.e. the person had a need in this domain in the last month), then ask the questions in Sections 2 to 4 on the same page.

Section 2

The purpose of this section is to record information about the current level of support for this domain from friends or family during the last month. If the interviewee has mentioned friends' names or family members, then personalise the question, but try not to exclude discussion of other people who may be helping. For example, "Does your Mum, or any other relative, help you to keep clean and tidy? How about friends?" would personalise Section 2 of self-care and presentation.

The rating indicates the level of help received, and anchor points are provided for guiding the rating of level of help. Note that what is being rated is the interviewee's perception of level of help; if they replied "My Dad nags me to tidy up, but I just ignore him" for the domain of looking after the home, then this would be rated as 0.

Try to avoid commenting on the reported level of support, because this could be perceived as either critical or patronising. It may be that help with different items is provided by different people. Do not ask how much help they feel that they need from friends or relatives.

Section 3   .

The purpose of this section is to gain information about the current and required level of support from local services over the last month. The two parts are best asked separately. As with Section 2, try to personalise the questions by being specific about local services. For example, "Do you talk to the nurses here when you feel sad? Anyone else here?" would be appropriate questions when interviewing a day patient at a day centre.

As with Section 2, rating involves considering the perceived effectiveness of an intervention. For example, if the person is on medication which is regularly reviewed, but reports that it does not help symptoms at all, then rate help received for psychotic symptoms as 0. The examples with each rating are meant to show the type of intervention which will constitute a low, medium or high level of help – what is being rated, however, is the level of perceived help.

The second part of Section 3 asks about the interviewee's perception of his or her need for help. Try to emphasise the word 'need', rather than asking how much help the person would like from local services. Note that the question is not asking how much extra help is needed. Use the same rating scale as for the first question in this section. A rating of 0 would indicate that the interviewee perceives no need for help from local services. When the same rating is given for the two questions in Section 3, this indicates the appropriate level of support from local services. When the rating is higher for the second question, this suggests the existence of unmet need.

Section 4

The purpose of this section is twofold:

(a)   To record any information given by the user that is not captured by the ratings, such as what help they would like in the future. This is only to be completed during the user interview.
(b)   To write action plans, which record what will be done (e.g. further assessment, specified intervention), who will do it and when the plan will be reviewed. This is completed by the member of staff.

Recording CAN–C assessments

CAN–C ratings can be recorded directly in the boxes on the form. Alternatively, three summary score sheets are shown in Appendix 3, which can be used to record an assessment using the CAN–C. These summary sheets are shorter and more suitable for case notes than a complete CAN–C. The CAN–C complete assessment summary sheet records a staff and user assessment of need, and the staff and user assessment summary sheets record individual assessments by the staff or the user. Each summary sheet allows the recording of summary variables: total number of met (need rating 1) and unmet (need rating 2) needs, the total number of needs (i.e. the sum of met and unmet needs), total level of help received from informal and formal sources, and total level of help needed from formal sources. In adding up these totals, always count a 9 (not known) as 0. Completing these extra boxes involves analysis of the data collected during assessment. If all that is required is a record of the assessment, then the extra boxes do not have to be completed. A record of the views of the user and any action plans will also need to be kept, for example on the back of the summary score sheet.

Using information from a CAN–C assessment

CAN–C assessment information can be used for at least two purposes:

(a)   CAN–C data can be used at the level of the individual user, by providing a baseline measure of level of need, or for charting changes in the user over time. For example, one approach would be to use the CAN–C routinely in initial assessments of new service users, to identify the range of domains in which they are likely to require further assessment and (possibly) help or treatment.
(b)   CAN–C data can be used for auditing and developing an individual service. For example, to investigate:

(i) the impact on needs of providing an intervention for a group of service users, by looking at changes across this group;

(ii) case load dependency for different workers;

(iii) whether enough users have unmet needs in the domain of Benefits to make it worthwhile for a community mental health team to employ a welfare benefits advisor.

6 Using the Camberwell Assessment of Need – Research version (CAN–R)

The Camberwell Assessment of Need – Research version (CAN–R) is intended for use as an outcome measure for research purposes, and is shown in Appendix 4, with summary score sheets in Appendix 5. It may be photocopied freely for your use.

The CAN–R has four sections for each domain, and is completed separately by the staff and service user. Section 1 assesses the need rating (no need, met need, unmet need or not known) for the domain. The purpose of Section 1 is twofold. First, to assess whether there is a need in the domain, and whether effective help is already being given. Second, to decide whether further questions about this domain are necessary. Section 2 assesses the amount of help from informal sources (friends, relatives, etc.). Section 3 assesses the amount of help given by and needed from formal services. For all ratings, anchor points and rating guidelines are provided. Section 4 records whether users are getting the right type of help for their problems and (in the user interview only) whether they are satisfied with the amount of help that they are receiving. It therefore differs from the CAN–C in that it assesses satisfaction, and does not record qualitative information on the user's perspective or the action plan.

The CAN–R assesses 22 domains of health and social needs.

1 Accommodation
2 Food
3 Looking after the home
4 Self-care
5 Daytime activities
6 Physical health
7 Psychotic symptoms
8 Information on condition and treatment
9 Psychological distress
10 Safety to self
11 Safety to others
12 Alcohol
13 Drugs
14 Company
15 Intimate relationships
16 Sexual expression
17 Child care
18 Basic education
19 Telephone
20 Transport

21   Money

22   Benefits

Questions are asked about each domain, to identify:

(a)   Whether a need or problem is present in that domain. A need is met if there is currently not a problem in the domain, but a problem would exist if it were not for the help provided (i.e. they are getting effective help). A need is unmet if there is currently a problem in the domain (whether or not any help is currently being provided).

(b)   Whether the need is met or unmet.

(c)   How much help the user is currently receiving from informal (friends, family, etc.) or formal sources, and how much help he or she needs.

(d)   Whether the user is getting the right type of help for his or her problem and (in the user interview only) whether he or she is satisfied with the amount of help that he or she is receiving.

At the end of an assessment, therefore, it will be possible to say how many needs the user has from these 22 domains, what help he or she is currently receiving and what help is needed, along with some information on satisfaction with care.

Each CAN–R can be used to record the perceptions of the staff and the user. One-page summary sheets are provided in Appendix 5, which reduce the research data to be stored.

An assessment using the CAN–R involves an interviewer asking an interviewee questions about each of 22 domains. The interviewer should be a professional with some knowledge of the difficulties which can be involved in interviewing people with SMI, such as impaired concentration, disorganisation and psychotic symptoms. The interviewer should also be familiar with issues relating to safety and confidentiality, as discussed by Parkman & Bixby (1996).

Administration of the CAN–R

The interviewee may be the user or a member of staff (e.g. the keyworker). If the user is being interviewed, administration involves the interviewer going through the CAN–R, asking the user about each domain in turn. If a member of staff is the interviewee, this may involve the member of staff filling in the CAN–R, or may involve them being interviewed by a trained research interviewer.

Whoever is being interviewed, it is important that it is their views which are assessed. Specifically, there are no 'right' or 'wrong' answers. So, for example, the staff members should give their own views about the users' needs, rather than what they think the users' views are.

The purpose of the interview should be explained to the interviewee. For the user, this explanation might take the form, "I'd like to go through this questionnaire with you, which covers a whole range of areas of life in which people can have difficulties. I'll go through each of these areas in turn, and ask about any problems you have had in the last month. Is that okay?" Time should be allowed for questions, and to ensure that the assessment is not rushed. A typical CAN–R assessment should take 10 minutes for the staff, and 15 minutes for the user, but this will be affected by the number of needs identified and characteristics of the interviewee. For example, if the user has difficulties with concentration, then a break may be needed during the interview.

Each of the 22 domains is assessed, in the order shown. Each domain comprises four sections. For each domain, care should be taken to ensure that the correct column (staff or user) is completed.

Section 1

Suggested opening questions are given in italics for each domain. Where necessary, follow-up questions can be asked, with the goal of establishing (a) whether the user experiences any problems in this domain; and (b) if the user does experience problems, is he or she getting effective help. On the basis of the interviewee's responses, a need rating is made:

0 = no serious problem   (no need)
1 = no/moderate problem due to help given   (met need)
2 = serious problem   (unmet need)
9 = not known

The need rating is made using the following algorithm:

If the interviewee does not know or does not want to answer questions on this domain then rate **9** (not known)

otherwise

If a serious problem is present (regardless of cause, or whether any help is being given or not) then rate **2** (unmet need)

otherwise

If there is no serious problem because of help given then rate **1** (met need)

otherwise

Rate **0** (no need)

Note Just because there is currently no problem, the need rating is not automatically 0. For example, a person with diabetes who is physically well because of the prescribed insulin would be rated as 1 (met need) for physical health.

Note A need can exist for a variety of reasons. For example, a person with a psychotic illness may currently be unable to do his or her shopping because of a sprained ankle. He or she should be rated as having a need (i.e. need rating 1 or 2) in the Food domain, even though this need is not related to his or her psychiatric condition.

For each domain, anchor points for the need ratings can be referred to in the CAN–R. However, the difference between rating 1 and 2 can be a matter of judgement. The goal is to differentiate between problems which are current and severe and those which are ameliorated by help, but there may still be a blurred boundary where the user is receiving help which only partly addresses his or her difficulties. Be guided by the interviewee's response – does he or she see the problem as current and severe (need rating 2), or under control with the help that the user is getting (need rating 1)?

For some of the 22 domains, there are some specific issues in Section 1 which have been found to require clarification.

1   Accommodation

If a person is currently in hospital and does not have a home to be discharged to, the need rating should be 1. If a person is currently in hospital and does have an appropriate home to be discharged to, the need rating should be 0 (this is an example of overmet need, which the CAN–R does not assess).

2 Food

A need is present if the person is not getting an adequate diet, due to difficulties with shopping, storage and/or cooking of food, or because inadequate or culturally inappropriate food is being provided (e.g. by a hospital ward). However, if the problem is primarily due to difficulties with budgeting then this should be rated under the domain of Money, and the Food rating should be 0.

3 Looking after the home

This domain concerns difficulties in maintaining the living environment, whether this is a hostel room or an independent home. It may not be possible for staff to rate this if the person is homeless, but the user may be able to state whether he or she believes that it would be a problem if he or she had a home.

4 Self-care

This domain refers to personal hygiene, and does not include untidiness or bizarre appearance.

5 Daytime activities

If the user is unable to occupy him- or herself during the day without help, then he or she has a need in this domain. Help given might include sheltered employment, attending a day centre, or activities with friends and relatives. If the primary problem is loneliness rather than boredom then this should be rated under the domain of Company.

6 Physical health

Physical side-effects of medication should be considered, as well as any acute or chronic medical or dental condition.

7 Psychotic symptoms

When asking the user about this domain particular care should be taken to record his or her perceptions. For example, a user who denies hearing voices and having problems with thoughts, and states that the depot injection is to keep him or her calm, should be rated as 0 (no need).

8 Information

This should include information about local service provision, as well as information about the user's specific condition.

9 Psychological distress

This should include depression and anxiety, regardless of the cause.

10 Safety to self

Risk due to severe self-neglect or vulnerability to exploitation should also be rated, as well as risk of suicide and self-harm.

11 Safety to others

Inadvertent risks (e.g. fire risk due to careless use of cigarettes) should be included, as well as risk of deliberate violence.

16 Sexual expression

This includes difficulties due to medication side-effects, as well as a lack of safe sex practices and inadequate contraception.

20 Transport

A need should be rated if a person is unable to use public transport for physical or psychological reasons.

21 Money

This refers to ability to cope with the available amount of money. If the user says that he or she does not have enough money, this should be assessed in the domain of Benefits.

If the rating is 0 or 9 go on to the next domain on the following page. If the rating is 1 or 2 (i.e. the person had a need in this domain in the last month), then ask the questions in Sections 2 to 4 on the same page.

Section 2

The purpose of this section is to record information about the current level of support for this domain from friends or family during the last month. If the interviewee has mentioned friends' names or family members, then personalise the question, but try not to exclude discussion of other people who may be helping. For example, "Does your Mum, or any other relative, help you to keep clean and tidy? How about friends?" would personalise Section 2 of self-care and presentation.

The rating indicates the level of help received, and anchor points are provided for guiding the rating of level of help. Note that what is being rated is the interviewee's perception of level of help; if they replied "My Dad nags me to tidy up, but I just ignore him" for the domain of looking after the home, then this would be rated as 0.

Try to avoid commenting on the reported level of support, because this could be perceived as either critical or patronising. It may be that help with different items is provided by different people. Do not ask how much help they feel that they need from friends or relatives.

Section 3

The purpose of this section is to gain information about the current and required level of support from local services over the last month. The two parts are best asked separately. As with Section 2, try to personalise the questions by being specific about local services. For example, "Do you talk to the nurses here when you feel sad? Anyone else here?" would be appropriate questions when interviewing a day patient at a day centre.

As with Section 2, rating involves considering the perceived effectiveness of an intervention. For example, if the person is on medication which is regularly reviewed, but reports that it does not help

24

symptoms at all, then rate help received for psychotic symptoms as 0. The examples with each rating are meant to show the type of intervention which will constitute a low, medium or high level of help – what is being rated, however, is the level of perceived help.

The second part of Section 3 asks about the interviewee's perception of his or her need for help. Try to emphasise the word 'need', rather than asking how much help the person would like from local services. Note that the question is not asking how much extra help is needed. Use the same rating scale as for the first question in this section. A rating of 0 would indicate that the interviewee perceives no need for help from local services. When the same rating is given for the two questions in Section 3, this indicates the appropriate level of support from local services. When the rating is higher for the second question, this suggests the existence of unmet need.

Section 4

The purpose of this section is to rate the interviewee's perception of the appropriateness and effectiveness of interventions. It can be difficult to distinguish between the two questions in this section, but it should be that sometimes different ratings are given for the two questions. The first question asks about the appropriateness of current interventions – do they think that different help should be given? The second question asks (the user only) about their satisfaction with the amount of help given – do they that think more help should be given? Staff are not asked this question because it could be seen as critical. This section is intended to identify when the person feels that either the wrong type of help is being offered, or not enough of the right type of help is being offered.

Recording CAN–R assessments

CAN–R ratings can be recorded directly in the boxes on the form. Alternatively, three summary score sheets are shown in Appendix 5, which can be used to record an assessment using the CAN–R. These summary sheets are shorter and easier to store than a complete CAN–R. The CAN–R complete assessment summary sheet records a staff and user assessment of need, and the staff and user assessment summary sheets record individual assessments by the staff or the user. Each summary sheet allows the recording of summary variables: total number of met (need rating 1) and unmet (need rating 2) needs; the total number of needs (i.e. the sum of met and unmet needs); total level of help received from informal and formal sources; total level of help needed from formal sources; and total level of satisfaction with type and amount of help. In adding up these totals, always count a 9 (not known) as 0. Completing these extra boxes involves analysis of the data collected during assessment. If all that is required is a record of the assessment, then the extra boxes do not have to be completed.

Using information from a CAN–R assessment

CAN–R assessment information is used as an outcome measure for research purposes, such as evaluating the impact on needs of two different types of mental health services (Leese et al, 1998), or investigating why staff and service user perceptions about need differ (Slade et al, 1996).

In research studies, comparisons between different data sets can only be made if there is a standard approach to data presentation and analysis. The approach outlined below should be followed in the initial analysis of any CAN data, with more complex analysis, if required, performed subsequently. The table below gives six summary scores, and suggests a convention that can be adopted for naming the variables if you use a software package such as SPSS (Statistical Package for the Social Sciences) for analysis. The maximum value of any variable is 22.

Summary score	Suggested variable name	
	User rating	Staff rating
Total number of met needs[1]	umet	smet
Total number of unmet needs[2]	uunmet	sunmet
Total number of needs[3]	unumneed	snumneed

1. The number of need ratings of 1 (met need) for the 22 domains.
2. The number of need ratings of 2 (unmet need) for the 22 domains.
3. The number of need ratings of 1 or 2 (met or unmet need) for the 22 domains (i.e. the sum of the total number of met and unmet needs).

Staff and user responses can be compared using Cohen's kappa coefficient or percentage agreement on either the presence of a need (i.e. need rating 1 or 2) or the precise need rating. One measure of the extent of overall agreement can be found by subtracting the staff from the user assessments of total (unumneed – snumneed), met (umet – smet) or unmet (sunmet – uunmet) needs.

Further analysis might compare the percentage of all needs which are met for users (umet/ unumneed) and staff (smet/snumneed), and investigate the total and mean scores for informal and formal care received, and formal care needed.

7 Training for the CAN

The CAN–R, CAN–C and CANSAS can normally be used without any formal training by mental health professionals. Each version contains a page outlining how to rate responses, and in the CAN–R and CAN–C every rating has anchor points for guidance. Reading through the CAN–R or CAN–C will give the rater a good overview of the approach used, and a relatively good assessment can be expected from the first use. The main improvement in subsequent assessments is likely to be in the time taken for assessment, which will reduce as familiarity with the questionnaire increases.

There will, however, be times when some training in the use of the CAN is appropriate. This might be for several reasons. The length (of the CAN–R or CAN–C) or complexity (of the CANSAS) may appear daunting, particularly if staff are not familiar with using assessment schedules. If the CANSAS or CAN–C is being introduced into routine clinical practice, there may be some resistance from staff, in which case training may serve to reduce apprehension, increase motivation and generate commitment from staff. Alternatively, it may be important to maximise inter-rater reliability from the outset.

This chapter provides an outline of a half-day training session which has been run several times by PRiSM. The goal of this training is both to educate participants about the approach taken to assessing need, and to give practice in rating the CAN–R. It can be easily modified as required for the CAN–C or CANSAS.

Each participant will need the following handouts:

1 programme for the day (written by trainer)
1 CAN–R (Appendix 4)
1 practice vignette (Appendix 6)
5 full vignettes (Appendix 6)
1 complete assessment summary sheet for each full vignette (Appendix 5)

The trainer will need an overhead projector, overhead pen and six overheads:

'Issues to consider' (Appendix 6)
CAN–R cover (Appendix 4)
CAN–R contents page (Appendix 4)
'Safety to self' assessment page (Appendix 4)
'Section 1' (Appendix 6)
'Sections 2 & 3' (Appendix 6)

The following programme comprises timings for the training session, together with notes for the trainer. The length of the training session can be adjusted as required.

Introduction to the CAN–R (30 minutes)

The goal is to introduce participants to the notion of need (as distinct from service response), and to give an outline of how to rate the CAN–R.

Circulate programme for the day

- Introductions of participants and trainer, if appropriate
- Clarify logistics – toilets, break times, etc.
- Brief introduction to purpose of the day – to learn about how to use the CAN
- Stress that this is not a lecture, and encourage participants to ask questions

Put up overhead titled 'Issues to consider'

- Outline what a need is
- Everyone has needs, which impact on quality of life
- Needs can be met, unmet or overmet
- Staff and mental health service users can differ in their perceptions about need
- Services should be provided on the basis of need

Put up overhead of CAN–R cover

- Introduce the CAN–R
- Brief history – developed at Institute of Psychiatry, first released 1994, research, clinical and short versions
- What will it be used for locally (e.g. 'to assess the needs of patients in our study')

Put up overhead of CAN–R contents page

- Introduce the 22 domains assessed using the CAN–R
- The domains span physical, psychological and social problem areas
- Every domain is assessed in the same way, so assessment is not as daunting as it might appear
- Goal of today is to give confidence in rating, and to ensure agreement between raters

Distribute CAN–R and put up overhead of 'Safety to self' page from the CAN–R

- Ask participants to find domain 10 in the CAN–R
- Introduce a typical page from the CAN–R, stressing that they are all structured in the same way
- Purpose of page is to record assessment of problems with suicide risk or other dangers
- Jargon has been avoided where possible (e.g. 'suicidal ideation')
- First thing to notice is that there are two columns, for separate ratings by staff and user, which are carried out in separate interviews
- It is acceptable for there to be differences between staff and user ratings

Put up overhead titled 'Section 1'

- Introduce purpose of Section 1 – to assess whether there is a problem with this area
- Use trigger questions (in italics in the CAN–R) to get into the topic
- Does it measure need? (yes)
- Does it measure existence of intervention? (no)

- Does it measure effectiveness of intervention? (yes, as perceived by respondent)
- **Principle:** always rate the response of the interviewee. Clarification is acceptable, judgement by rater is not
- What is an intervention? (any help received from either formal or informal sources)
- How to rate when there is an intervention but no perceived need? (0 – the CAN–R does not measure overmet need)
- How to rate when there is a totally effective intervention? (1)
- How to rate when there is a partially effective intervention (1 or 2, depending on interviewee's perception of whether the problem is still serious)
- **Principle:** the anchor points are just guidelines for rating
- How to rate when there is a totally ineffective intervention (2)

Put up overhead titled 'Sections 2 & 3'

- Section 2 measures help received from informal sources – friends, relatives, neighbours, etc.
- Section 3 measures help received and needed from formal services
- Level of help is being rated, with anchor points as guidance
- What about when the intervention is perceived as not helping? (rate 0, even if help given is an anchor point for a higher rating)
- Difference between help given and needed – stress that the interviewee's response is recorded, whether realistic or not
- Section 4 – what is the difference? (type versus amount of help)

Practice vignette (30 minutes)

Distribute practice vignette

- Goal is to have a first attempt at rating the CAN–R – to help, the expected ratings are given
- Split into pairs, and decide who will be Jeanette and who the rater
- Jeanette reads the role-play instructions, and the rater looks at 'Safety to self' and 'Safety to others' sections in the CAN–R (domains 10 and 11)
- Emphasise that ratings are to be done in the 'User' column
- Role-play doing the assessment of Jeanette on these two topics
- Stop the role-play (after 10 minutes), and discuss scoring in pairs
- Swap roles (after 5 minutes), so rater becomes Dr Jones and Jeanette becomes rater
- Role-play assessment of Dr Jones, emphasising that ratings are to be in the 'Staff' column
- Stop the role-play (after 10 minutes) and discuss scoring in pairs (for five minutes)

Feedback on practice vignette (20 minutes)

Put up overhead of 'Safety to self' assessment page from the CAN–R

Go through the page, scoring on the overhead. Discuss both pages as a large group, highlighting and addressing issues. It is important to encourage people to ask when they do not understand. If somebody says, "I don't understand how to..." then use it as a teaching opportunity by saying to the group, "So it isn't clear how to...".

Full vignette 1 (60 minutes)

Distribute full vignette and complete assessment summary sheet

The rest of the programme can be tailored to individual requirements. Normally 60 minutes is necessary for each full vignette. Each vignette will require one complete assessment summary sheet, with the CAN–R used for reference. Different ways of running this part include:

(a) In pairs, role-play the interviewee (user or staff) with the other one rating. This approach is useful for gaining familiarity with the CAN–R, and generates most questions.

(b) Work through the vignette on your own, rating as you go. This approach is useful for a group lacking confidence in using assessment schedules.

(c) The trainer role-plays the assessment with a volunteer, while all participants rate from responses made. This approach is useful for participants seeing 'how to do it'.

8 Frequently asked questions

What is the CAN?

The Camberwell Assessment of Need (CAN) is a family of questionnaires for assessing the wide range of problems which can be experienced by a person with severe mental health problems. It covers 22 different areas of life, and can be used to assess the perceptions of the service users, their carers, and the members of staff working with them (i.e. mental health professionals). Three versions are available – a clinical version (CAN–C), a research version (CAN–R) and a short version (CANSAS).

What is the CANSAS?

The Camberwell Assessment of Need (CANSAS) is a short (one-page) assessment which summarises whether a person with mental health problems has difficulties in 22 different areas of life, and whether they are currently receiving any effective help with these difficulties. CANSAS is designed to be used in routine clinical work or as an outcome measure in research studies. A copy of the CANSAS for photocopying is given in Appendix 1, and directions for using it are given in Chapter 4.

What is the CAN–C?

The Camberwell Assessment of Need – Clinical version (CAN–C) is an in-depth assessment of whether people with mental health problems have difficulties in 22 different areas of life. It assesses what sort of help they are currently receiving for these difficulties, and how much help they need. It also provides space for recording their views about what help should be offered, and for a care plan. The CAN–C is designed to be used in clinical work where a detailed assessment is required. A copy of the CAN–C for photocopying is given in Appendix 2, summary score sheets in Appendix 3 and directions for using it are given in Chapter 5.

What is the CAN–R?

The Camberwell Assessment of Need – Research version (CAN–R) is an in-depth assessment of whether people with mental health problems have difficulties in 22 different areas of life. It assesses what sort of help they are currently receiving for these difficulties, how much help they need, and their satisfaction with the help given. CAN–R is designed to be used in research studies. A copy of the CAN–R for photocopying is given in Appendix 4, summary score sheets in Appendix 5 and directions for using it are given in Chapter 6.

How do I score the need rating if the user's perception is that there is no problem, but they are receiving help?

When making a user rating, always record the user's perspective, even if this appears irrational or inconsistent with what is known about them. If they say that there is no problem, prompt to see if they are receiving any help in that area. If they are, ask them what the help is for. If they acknowledge that the help prevents the problem, then rate 1 (i.e. no problem because of continuing intervention). If they say that the help is not connected with the problem, code 0. Three examples to illustrate this:

(a) Psychotic symptoms   The user says they do not hear voices, but on prompting they report that they have a fortnightly depot antipsychotic injection. Ask them what the injection is for. If they know it is to prevent their symptoms recurring, rate 1; if they think it is for an unrelated reason, rate 0; if they do not know why they receive the injection, go back and ask again if they have a problem in this area. If they say there is no problem, rate 0.

(b) Safety to self   In the past month the user took an overdose and was seen by the duty psychiatrist in casualty. No further follow-up was arranged and the user maintains that they were not trying to kill themselves. Rate 0.

(c) Accommodation and food   The user lives in the parental home and has food provided there. They report 'no problem' with either domain. Prompt to ask why they live at home and ask if they could live independently. Rate 0 if they choose to live at home and say they could manage independently.

How do I score the need rating if the interviewee says there is still a need even though an intervention is being offered?

A rating of 1 indicates met need, whether fully met (an intervention totally removes the problem) or partially met (there is still a moderate problem despite the intervention). A rating of 2 indicates unmet need and can be rated in the presence or absence of an intervention if a serious problem exists. If the interviewee perceives the intervention as totally ineffective, rate 2. If they perceive the intervention as reducing the problem to a moderate ('subclinical') level, rate 1. If in doubt, ask the interviewee whether they see the problem as moderate or serious.

In CAN-R or CAN-C, how do I rate Section 3 if a service has been offered but the user has refused it?

Section 3 relates to actual receipt of help from formal services. If a service has been offered but they have refused it, then they are not receiving any help and are rated 0 (no help). The questions asking about satisfaction with type and amount of help received might inform understanding of this situation. Perhaps they have refused help because they perceive it to be of the wrong sort.

Are all the domains meant to be areas which clinical teams should be addressing? How do I rate the domain if I would not offer an intervention for that particular problem?

The 22 domains were widely agreed to be relevant domains of need, although any particular team might only address some of these. Irrespective of whether the team would address this problem, the problem should be rated if it exists. For some items (such as accommodation) one type of help that might be offered is a referral to a more appropriate agency.

What if I think that you should have included other domains, such as spiritual needs? Can I add them in?

You can add them in, but be aware that the reliability and validity of any extra domains have not been established. Also, do not substitute them for existing domains, or include them in the recommended scoring methods.

Is it acceptable to combine different sources of information in a single CAN assessment?

This is not recommended. For example, there is often a disparity between staff and user ratings. Therefore, it is likely that using different sources to make a single rating will lose the information about where there are disagreements. This is why each assessment can be recorded separately.

Can I just do user or staff ratings?

The CAN may be used for only user or only staff ratings, and summary score sheets are provided for this purpose. However, research indicates that staff and service users do not rate identically, so information is lost when only one perspective is assessed. One of the strengths of the CAN is that it does identify differences in staff and user assessments of need. Further discussion of this can be found in Slade *et al* (1996).

How do I compare staff and user ratings of need?

For clinical purposes, this is best done by negotiation between the member of staff and the service user. This is discussed in Slade (1994). For research purposes, use the method in Slade *et al* (1996).

What client groups can I use the CAN with?

The CAN was developed and tested with adults who had a clinical diagnosis of a major psychotic disorder and were receiving help from mental health services either in hospital or the community. This is therefore the client group for which the CAN described in this book is most suitable.

Other versions of the CAN are being developed for use with people with learning disabilities (CANDID) and older adults (CANE). Please contact PRiSM at the Institute of Psychiatry for further details.

What sample size do I need for a study using the CAN?

To decide on a sample size you need to decide:

(a)   the power (e.g. 0.8);
(b)   the significance level (e.g. 0.05);
(c)   the level of difference you wish to detect (or the difference you think will arise);
(d)   typical levels of variation (standard deviations) for continuous variables.

Values for (a) and (b) must be selected by the researcher, whereas values for (c) and (d) should, ideally, be estimated for a specific setting by a pilot study. However, to give some idea of the likely levels of variation, some typical values are given below (user ratings). The numbers that would be required to detect differences at these levels, with significance 0.05 and power 0.8, are also shown.

Continuous variables	Group means		Within group variation	Number required
	Group 1	Group 2	(s.d.)	per group
Number of met needs (range 0–22)	4.0	5.0	2.0	63
Number of unmet needs (range 0–22)	1.5	2.5	2.5	99

Presence/absence variables	Group 1	Group 2	Number required per group
Psychotic symptoms	65%	80%	151
Accommodation	30%	45%	176
Drugs	5%	10%	474

Relevant references are Altman (1982) and Campbell & Machin (1993, p.110).

Is the CAN available in other languages?

Yes. As part of an international study, translations into Danish, Dutch, Italian and Spanish have been completed, using focus groups and back-translations to ensure cross-cultural validity. The CAN has also been translated into French, German, Greek, Swedish and Turkish. There has been interest expressed in translating the CAN into Japanese, Norwegian and Portugese. Requests for further information about translations should be sent to PRiSM, Insititute of Psychiatry.

What do I do if my question has not been answered?

Write with your question to: Section of Community Psychiatry (PRiSM), Institute of Psychiatry, Denmark Hill, London SE5 8AF, England.

References

Altman, D. G. (1982) How large a sample? In *Statistics in Practice* (eds S. M. Gore & D. G. Altman), pp. 6–8. London: British Medical Association.

Baker, R. & Hall, J. (1988) REHAB: A new assessment instrument for chronic psychiatric patients. *Schizophrenia Bulletin*, **14**, 97–111.

Bradshaw, J. (1972) A taxonomy of social need. In *Problems and Progress in Medical Care: Essays on Current Research* (ed. G. McLachlan) (7th Series), pp. 71–82. London: Oxford University Press.

Brewin, C., Wing, J., Mangen, S., et al (1987) Principles and practice of measuring needs in the long-term mentally ill: the MRC Needs for Care Assessment. *Psychological Medicine*, **17**, 971–981.

——, ——, ——, et al (1988) Needs for care among the long-term mentally ill: a report from the Camberwell High Contact Survey. *Psychological Medicine*, **18**, 457–468.

Campbell, M. J. & Machin, D. (1993) *Medical Statistics: A Commonsense Approach*. New York: Wiley.

Carter, M., Crosby, C., Geerthuis, S., et al (1996) Developing reliability in client-centred mental health needs assessment. *Journal of Mental Health*, **5**, 233–243.

Glover, G., Robin, E., Emami, J., et al (1998) A needs index for mental health care. *Social Psychiatry and Psychiatric Epidemiology*, **33**, 89–96.

Hogg, L. & Marshall, M. (1992) Can we measure need in the homeless mentally ill? Using the MRC Needs for Care Assessment in hostels for the homeless. *Psychological Medicine*, **22**, 1027–1034.

Holloway, F. (1993) Need in community psychiatry: a consensus is required. *Psychiatric Bulletin*, **18**, 321–323.

Jarman, B. (1983) Identification of underprivileged areas. *British Medical Journal*, **286**, 1705–1709.

Johnson, S., Thornicroft, G., Phelan, M., et al (1996) Assessing needs for mental health services. In *Mental Health Outcome Measures* (eds G. Thornicroft & M. Tansella), pp. 217–226. Berlin: Springer.

Leese, M., Johnson, S., Slade, M., et al (1998) User perspective on needs and satisfaction with mental health services. PRiSM Psychosis Study 8. *British Journal of Psychiatry*, **173**, 409–415.

LeSage, A., Mignolli, G., Faccincani, C., et al (1991) Standardised assessment of the needs for care in a cohort of patients with schizophrenic psychoses. *Psychological Medicine*, **19** (suppl.), 426–431.

Marshall, M. (1994) How should we measure need? *Philosophy, Psychiatry and Psychology*, **1**, 27–36.

Maslow, A. (1954) *Motivation and Personality*. New York: Harper and Row.

O'Leary, D. & Webb, M. (1996) The needs for care assessment: a longitudinal approach. *Psychiatric Bulletin*, **20**, 134–136.

Parkman, S. & Bixby, S. (1996) Community interviewing: experiences and recommendations. *Psychiatric Bulletin*, **20**, 72–74.

Phelan, M., Slade, M., Thornicroft, G., et al (1995) The Camberwell Assessment of Need: the validity and reliability of an instrument to assess the needs of people with severe mental illness. *British Journal of Psychiatry*, **167**, 589–595.

Pryce, I. G., Griffiths, R. D., Gentry, R. M., et al (1993) How important is the assessment of social skills in current long-stay patients? An evaluation of clinical response to needs for assessment, treatment and care in long-stay psychiatric in-patient population. *British Journal of Psychiatry*, **162**, 498–502.

Slade, M. (1994) Needs assessment. *British Journal of Psychiatry*, **165**, 293–296.

——, Phelan, M., Thornicroft, G., et al (1996) The Camberwell Assessment of Need (CAN): comparison of assessments by staff and patients of the needs of the severely mentally ill. *Social Psychiatry and Psychiatric Epidemiology*, **31**, 109–113.

Stevens, A. & Gabbay, J. (1991) Needs assessment needs assessment… *Health Trends*, **23**, 20–23.

Thornicroft, G. (1991) Social deprivation and rates of treated mental disorder: developing statistical models to predict psychiatric service utilisation. *British Journal of Psychiatry*, **158**, 475–484.

Van Haaster, I., LeSage, A., Cyr, M., et al (1994) Problems and needs for care of patients suffering from severe mental illness. *Social Psychiatry and Psychiatric Epidemiology*, **29**, 141–148.

Appendix 1

Camberwell Assessment of Need Short Appraisal Schedule (CANSAS)

How to use the CANSAS

What is the CANSAS?

The CANSAS is a tool for the comprehensive assessment of the needs of people with severe mental health problems. It is designed for research and clinical use, in conjunction with Chapter 4. Interviewers will need to have experience of clinical assessment interviews, and reliability will be increased by using the training programme contained in Chapter 7.

How do I complete the CANSAS?

The CANSAS assesses problems during the last one month in 22 domains of life. This relatively short time span leads to a snapshot of the current situation. Assessment may involve an interview with a service user (the term used to cover patient/client/consumer – the person being assessed), a carer or a staff member who knows the user sufficiently well. It is important that the interviewee's reply is recorded directly, even if the interviewer disagrees with his or her view. User, staff and carer perceptions of need may differ, which is why they are recorded in separate columns.

Each assessment uses one column. Circle the letter indicating who is being assessed (U=user, S=staff, C=carer), and record the date and initials of the interviewer. Work down the column using the suggested questions (shown in italics) to open discussion on each domain. Supplementary questions should be asked where necessary, with the goal of establishing:

(a) whether the user has a serious problem in this domain; and
(b) if the user does have a serious problem, whether he or she is getting effective help.

On the basis of the interviewee's responses, a 'need rating' is made for the last month:

0 = no need (i.e. no serious problem)
1 = met need (i.e. no/moderate problem due to help given)
2 = unmet need (i.e. serious problem, whether or not help is given)
9 = not known

The need rating is made using the following guidelines:

- If a serious problem is present (regardless of cause, or whether or not any help is being given), then **rate 2** (unmet need).
- If there is no serious problem because help is being given (e.g. family support, sheltered housing, psychotherapy, medication), then **rate 1** (met need).
- If there are no problems in this area, then **rate 0** (no need).
- If the person being interviewed does not know or does not want to answer questions on this domain, then **rate 9** (not known).

Note

- Just because there is currently no problem, the need rating is not automatically 0. For example, a person with diabetes who is physically well because of the prescribed insulin would be rated as 1 (met need) for physical health.

- A need can exist for a variety of reasons. For example, a person with a psychotic illness may currently be unable to go shopping because of a sprained ankle. He or she should be rated as having a need (i.e. need rating 1 or 2) in the Food domain, even though this need is not related to his or her psychiatric condition.

- The CANSAS does not assess overmet need. For example, if a person was an in-patient for the last month, but has what he or she considers to be adequate accommodation outside of hospital, then accommodation should be rated as 0, even though he or she is currently being provided with hospital accommodation.

Camberwell Assessment of Need Short Appraisal Schedule

User/Client name	Need rating
	0 = no problem 2 = unmet need 1 = met need 9 = not known

	1	2	3	4
Assessment number				
Circle who is interviewed (U=User, S=Staff, C=Carer)	U / S / C	U / S / C	U / S / C	U / S / C
Date of assessment				
Initials of assessor				

		1	2	3	4
1	**Accommodation** *What kind of place do you live in?*				
2	**Food** *Do you get enough to eat?*				
3	**Looking after the home** *Are you able to look after your home?*				
4	**Self-care** *Do you have problems keeping clean and tidy?*				
5	**Daytime activities** *How do you spend your day?*				
6	**Physical health** *How well do you feel physically?*				
7	**Psychotic symptoms** *Do you ever hear voices or have problems with your thoughts?*				
8	**Information on condition and treatment** *Have you been given clear information about your medication?*				
9	**Psychological distress** *Have you recently felt very sad or low?*				
10	**Safety to self** *Do you ever have thoughts of harming yourself?*				
11	**Safety to others** *Do you think you could be a danger to other people's safety?*				
12	**Alcohol** *Does drinking cause you any problems?*				
13	**Drugs** *Do you take any drugs that aren't prescribed?*				
14	**Company** *Are you happy with your social life?*				
15	**Intimate relationships** *Do you have a partner?*				
16	**Sexual expression** *How is your sex life?*				
17	**Child care** *Do you have any children under 18?*				
18	**Basic education** *Any difficulty in reading, writing or understanding English?*				
19	**Telephone** *Do you know how to use a telephone?*				
20	**Transport** *How do you find using the bus, tube or train?*				
21	**Money** *How do you find budgeting your money?*				
22	**Benefits** *Are you getting all the money you are entitled to?*				

		1	2	3	4
A	Met needs – count the number of 1s in the column				
B	Unmet need – count the number of 2s in the column				
C	Total number of needs – add together A + B				

Appendix 2

Camberwell Assessment of Need –
Clinical version (CAN–C)

How to use the CAN–C

What is the CAN–C?

The CAN–C is a tool for the comprehensive assessment of the needs of people with severe mental health problems. It is designed for clinical use, in conjunction with Chapter 5. Interviewers will need to have experience of clinical assessment interviews, and reliability will be increased by using the training programme contained in Chapter 7.

How do I complete the CAN–C?

The CAN–C assesses problems during the last one month in 22 domains of life. This relatively short time span leads to a snapshot of the current situation. Assessment should comprise an interview where the member of staff records the views of the user (the term used to cover patient/client/consumer – the person being assessed) and then (separately) either an interview or self-completion to record the staff assessment. It is important that the user's response is recorded directly even if the interviewer disagrees with this view – user and staff perceptions of need do differ.

Each page contains four sections (each in a box). Use the suggested questions above Section 1 (shown in italics) to open discussion on each domain. Supplementary questions should be asked where necessary, with the goal of establishing:

(a) whether the user has a serious problem in this domain; and
(b) if the user does have a serious problem, whether he or she is getting effective help.

On the basis of the interviewee's responses, a *need rating* is made for the last month:

0 = no serious problem (i.e. no need)
1 = no/moderate problem due to help given (i.e. met need)
2 = serious problem (i.e. unmet need, whether or not help is given)
9 = not known

The need rating is made using the following guidelines:

- If a serious problem is present (regardless of cause, and whether or not any help is being given), then **rate 2**.
- If there is *no* serious problem *because* help is being given (e.g. family support, sheltered housing, psychotherapy, medication), then **rate 1**.
- If there are no problems in this area, then **rate 0**.
- If the person being interviewed does not know or does not want to answer questions on this domain, then **rate 9**.

If a need is not identified, then go on to the next domain. Sections 2–4 are only completed if a need is identified (i.e. need rating is 1 or 2). Section 2 assesses help received from informal sources (e.g.

friends, family, neighbours) and Section 3 the help received from formal sources (e.g. health, housing and social services). Section 3 also records the interviewee's perceptions of help needed, to allow undermet need to be identified. Section 4 records information about what help the user wants, and any action plan agreed between staff and user.

Note

- Just because there is currently no problem, the need rating is not automatically 0. For example a person with diabetes who is well because of the prescribed insulin would be rated as 1 for physical health.
- A need can exist for a variety of reasons. For example, a person with a psychotic illness may currently be unable to go shopping because of a sprained ankle. He or she should be rated as having a need (i.e. need rating 1 or 2) in the Food domain, even though this need is not related to his or her psychiatric condition.
- The CAN–C does not assess over-provision of services. For example, if a person was an inpatient for the last month, but has what he or she considers to be adequate accommodation outside hospital, then accommodation should be rated as 0, even though he or she is currently being provided with hospital accommodation.

Contents

1 Accommodation

What kind of place do you live in?
What sort of place is it?

Does the person lack a current place to stay?

Rating	Meaning	Example
0	No problem	Person does have an adequate home (even if in hospital currently)
1	No/moderate problem due to help given	Person is living in sheltered accommodation or hostel
2	Serious problem	Person is homeless, precariously housed, or home lacks basic facilities such as water and electricity
9	Not known	

If rated 0 or 9 go to next page

How much help with accommodation does the person receive from friends or relatives?

Rating	Meaning	Example
0	None	
1	Low help	Occasionally supplied with few pieces of furniture
2	Moderate help	Substantial help with improving accommodation, such as redecoration of flat
3	High help	Living with relative because own accommodation is unsatisfactory
9	Not known	

How much help with accommodation does the person *receive* from local services?

How much help with accommodation does the person *need* from local services?

Rating	Meaning	Example
0	None	
1	Low help	Minor decoration, address of housing agency
2	Moderate help	Major improvements, referral to housing agency
3	High help	Being rehoused, living in group home or hostel
9	Not known	

User's view of services required

Action(s)	By whom	Review date

2 Food

What kind of food do you eat?
Are you able to prepare your own meals and do your own shopping?

Does the person have difficulty in getting enough to eat?

Rating	Meaning	Example
0	No problem	Able to buy and prepare meals
1	No/moderate problem due to help given	Unable to prepare food and has meals provided
2	Serious problem	Very restricted diet, culturally inappropriate food
9	Not known	

If rated 0 or 9 go to next page

How much help with getting enough to eat does the person receive from friends or relatives?

Rating	Meaning	Example
0	None	
1	Low help	Meal provided weekly or less
2	Moderate help	Weekly help with shopping or meals provided more than weekly but not daily
3	High help	Meal provided daily
9	Not known	

How much help with getting enough to eat does the person *receive* from local services?

How much help with getting enough to eat does the person *need* from local services?

Rating	Meaning	Example
0	None	
1	Low help	1–4 meals a week provided, or assisted for one meal a day
2	Moderate help	More than 4 meals a week provided, or assisted for all meals
3	High help	All meals provided
9	Not known	

User's view of services required

Action(s) | By whom | Review date

3 Looking after the home

Are you able to look after your home?
Does anyone help you?

Does the person have difficulty looking after the home?

Rating	Meaning	Example
0	No problem	Home may be untidy but the person keeps it basically clean
1	No/moderate problem due to help given	Unable to look after home and has regular domestic help
2	Serious problem	Home is dirty and a potential health hazard
9	Not known	

If rated 0 or 9 go to next page

How much help with looking after the home does the person receive from friends or relatives?

Rating	Meaning	Example
0	None	
1	Low help	Prompts or helps tidy up or clean occasionally
2	Moderate help	Prompts or helps clean at least once a week
3	High help	Supervises the person more than once a week, washes all clothes and cleans the home
9	Not known	

How much help with looking after the home does the person *receive* from local services?

How much help with looking after the home does the person *need* from local services?

Rating	Meaning	Example
0	None	
1	Low help	Prompting by staff
2	Moderate help	Some assistance with household tasks
3	High help	Majority of household tasks done by staff
9	Not known	

User's view of services required

Action(s)	By whom	Review date

4   Self-care

Do you have problems keeping clean and tidy?
Do you ever need reminding? Who by?

Does the person have difficulty with self-care?

Rating	Meaning	Example
0	No problem	Appearance may be eccentric or untidy, but basically clean
1	No/moderate problem due to help given	Needs and gets help with self-care
2	Serious problem	Poor personal hygiene, smells
9	Not known	

If rated 0 or 9 go to next page

How much help with self-care does the person receive from friends or relatives?

Rating	Meaning	Example
0	None	
1	Low help	Occasionally prompt the person to change their clothes
2	Moderate help	Run the bath/shower and insist on its use, daily prompting
3	High help	Provide daily assistance with several aspects of care
9	Not known	

How much help with self-care does the person *receive* from local services?

How much help with self-care does the person *need* from local services?

Rating	Meaning	Example
0	None	
1	Low help	Occasional prompting
2	Moderate help	Supervise weekly washing
3	High help	Supervise several aspects of self-care, self-care skills programme
9	Not known	

User's view of services required

Action(s)

	By whom	Review date

5 Daytime activities

How do you spend your day?
Do you have enough to do?

Assessments

| User rating | Staff rating |

Does the person have difficulty with regular, appropriate daytime activities?

Rating	Meaning	Example
0	No problem	In full time employment, or adequately occupied with household/social activities
1	No/moderate problem due to help given	Unable to occupy self, so attending day centre
2	Serious problem	No employment of any kind and not adequately occupied with household/social activities
9	Not known	

If rated 0 or 9 go to next page

How much help does the person receive from friends or relatives in finding or keeping regular and appropriate daytime activities?

Rating	Meaning	Example
0	None	
1	Low help	Occasional advice about daytime activities
2	Moderate help	Has arranged daytime activities such as adult education or day centre attendance
3	High help	Daily help with arranging daytime activities
9	Not known	

How much help does the person *receive* from local services in finding or keeping regular and appropriate daytime activities?

How much help does the person *need* from local services in finding or keeping regular and appropriate daytime activities?

Rating	Meaning	Example
0	None	
1	Low help	Employment training/adult education
2	Moderate help	Sheltered employment daily. Day centre 2–4 days a week
3	High help	Attends day hospital or day centre daily
9	Not known	

User's view of services required

Action(s)	By whom	Review date

6   Physical health

How well do you feel physically?
Are you getting any treatment for physical problems from your doctor?

Assessments

User rating   Staff rating

Does the person have any physical disability or any physical illness?

Rating	Meaning	Example
0	No problem	Physically well
1	No/moderate problem due to help given	Physical ailment, such as high blood pressure, receiving appropriate treatment
2	Serious problem	Untreated physical ailment, including side-effects
9	Not known	

If rated 0 or 9 go to next page

How much help does the person receive from friends or relatives for physical health problems?

Rating	Meaning	Example
0	None	
1	Low help	Prompting to go to doctor
2	Moderate help	Accompanied to doctor
3	High help	Daily help with going to the toilet, eating or mobility
9	Not known	

How much help does the person *receive* from local services for physical health problems?

How much help does the person *need* from local services for physical health problems?

Rating	Meaning	Example
0	None	
1	Low help	Given dietary or family planning advice
2	Moderate help	Prescribed medication. Regularly seen by GP/nurse
3	High help	Frequent hospital appointments. Alterations to home
9	Not known	

User's view of services required

Action(s)

	By whom	Review date

7 Psychotic symptoms

Do you ever hear voices, or have problems with your thoughts?
Are you on any medication or injections? What is it for?

Assessments

User rating   Staff rating

Does the person have any psychotic symptoms?

Rating	Meaning	Example
0	No problem	No positive symptoms, not at risk from symptoms and not on medication
1	No/moderate problem due to help given	Symptoms helped by medication or other help
2	Serious problem	Currently has symptoms or at risk
9	Not known	

If rated 0 or 9 go to next page

How much help does the person receive from friends or relatives for these psychotic symptoms?

Rating	Meaning	Example
0	None	
1	Low help	Some sympathy and support
2	Moderate help	Carers involved in helping with coping strategies or medication compliance
3	High help	Constant supervision of medication, and help with coping strategies
9	Not known	

How much help does the person *receive* from local services for these psychotic symptoms?

How much help does the person *need* from local services for these psychotic symptoms?

Rating	Meaning	Example
0	None	
1	Low help	Medication reviewed thrice monthly or less, support group
2	Moderate help	Medication reviewed more than thrice monthly, structured psychological therapy
3	High help	Medication and 24-hour hospital care or crisis care at home
9	Not known	

User's view of services required

Action(s)

	By whom	Review date

8   Information on condition and treatment

Have you been given clear information about your medication or other treatment?
How helpful has the information been?

Has the person had clear verbal or written information about condition and treatment?

Rating	Meaning	Example
0	No problem	Has received and understood adequate information
1	No/moderate problem due to help given	Has not received or understood all information
2	Serious problem	Has received no information
9	Not known	

If rated 0 or 9 go to next page

How much help does the person receive from friends or relatives in obtaining such information?

Rating	Meaning	Example
0	None	
1	Low help	Has had some advice from friends or relatives
2	Moderate help	Given leaflets/factsheets or put in touch with self-help groups by friends or relatives
3	High help	Regular liaison with doctors or groups such as MIND, by friends or relatives
9	Not known	

How much help does the person *receive* from local services in obtaining such information?

How much help does the person *need* from local services in obtaining such information?

Rating	Meaning	Example
0	None	
1	Low help	Brief verbal or written information on illness/problem/treatment
2	Moderate help	Given details of self-help groups. Long verbal information sessions on drugs and alternative treatments.
3	High help	Has been given detailed written information or has had specific personal education
9	Not known	

User's view of services required

Action(s)	By whom	Review date

9 Psychological distress

Have you recently felt very sad or low?
Have you felt overly anxious or frightened?

Does the person suffer from current psychological distress?

Rating	Meaning	Example
0	No problem	Occasional or mild distress
1	No/moderate problem due to help given	Needs and gets ongoing support
2	Serious problem	Has expressed suicidal ideas during last month or has exposed themselves to serious danger
9	Not known	

If rated 0 or 9 go to next page

How much help does the person receive from friends or relatives for this distress?

Rating	Meaning	Example
0	None	
1	Low help	Some sympathy or support
2	Moderate help	Has opportunity at least weekly to talk about distress to friend or relative
3	High help	Constant support and supervision
9	Not known	

How much help does the person *receive* from local services for this distress?

How much help does the person *need* from local services for this distress?

Rating	Meaning	Example
0	None	
1	Low help	Assessment of mental state or occasional support
2	Moderate help	Specific psychological or social treatment for anxiety. Counselled by staff at least once a week
3	High help	24-hour hospital care or crisis care
9	Not known	

User's view of services required

Action(s)	By whom	Review date

10 Safety to self

Do you ever have thoughts of harming yourself, or actually harm yourself?
Do you put yourself in danger in other ways?

Assessments

User rating | Staff rating

Is the person a danger to him- or herself?

Rating	Meaning	Example
0	No problem	No suicidal thoughts
1	No/moderate problem due to help given	Suicide risk monitored by staff, receiving counselling
2	Serious problem	Distress affects life significantly, such as preventing person going out
9	Not known	

If rated 0 or 9 go to next page

How much help does the person receive from friends or relatives to reduce the risk of self-harm?

Rating	Meaning	Example
0	None	
1	Low help	Able to contact friends or relatives if feeling unsafe
2	Moderate help	Friends or relatives are usually in contact and are likely to know if feeling unsafe
3	High help	Friends or relatives in regular contact and are very likely to know and provide help if feeling unsafe
9	Not known	

How much help does the person *receive* from local services to reduce the risk of self-harm?

How much help does the person *need* from local services to reduce the risk of self-harm?

Rating	Meaning	Example
0	None	
1	Low help	Someone to contact when feeling unsafe
2	Moderate help	Staff check at least once a week, regular supportive counselling
3	High help	Daily supervision, in-patient care
9	Not known	

User's view of services required

Action(s) | By whom | Review date

11 Safety to others

Do you think you could be a danger to other people's safety?
Do you ever lose your temper and hit someone?

Is the person a current or potential risk to other people's safety?

Rating	Meaning	Example
0	No problem	No history of violence or threatening behaviour
1	No/moderate problem due to help given	At risk from alcohol misuse and receiving help
2	Serious problem	Recent violence or threats
9	Not known	

If rated 0 or 9 go to next page

How much help does the person receive from friends or relatives to reduce the risk that he or she might harm someone else?

Rating	Meaning	Example
0	None	
1	Low help	Help with threatening behaviour weekly or less
2	Moderate help	Help with threatening behaviour more than weekly
3	High help	Almost constant help with persistently threatening behaviour
9	Not known	

How much help does the person *receive* from local services to reduce the risk that he or she might harm someone else?

How much help does the person *need* from local services to reduce the risk that he or she might harm someone else?

Rating	Meaning	Example
0	None	
1	Low help	Check on behaviour weekly or less
2	Moderate help	Daily supervision
3	High help	Constant supervision. Anger management programme
9	Not known	

User's view of services required

Action(s)	By whom	Review date

12 Alcohol

Does drinking cause you any problems?
Do you wish you could cut down your drinking?

Does the person drink excessively, or have a problem controlling his or her drinking?

Rating	Meaning	Example
0	No problem	No problem with controlled drinking
1	No/moderate problem due to help given	Under supervision because of potential risk
2	Serious problem	Current drinking harmful or uncontrollable
9	Not known	

If rated 0 or 9 go to next page

How much help does the person receive from friends or relatives for this drinking?

Rating	Meaning	Example
0	None	
1	Low help	Told to cut down
2	Moderate help	Advised about Alcoholics Anonymous
3	High help	Daily monitoring of alcohol
9	Not known	

How much help does the person *receive* from local services for this drinking?

How much help does the person *need* from local services for this drinking?

Rating	Meaning	Example
0	None	
1	Low help	Told about risks
2	Moderate help	Given details of helping agencies
3	High help	Attends alcohol clinic, supervised withdrawal programme
9	Not known	

User's view of services required

Action(s)

	By whom	Review date

13 Drugs

Do you take any drugs that aren't prescribed?
Are there any drugs you would find hard to stop taking?

Does the person have problems with drug misuse?

Rating	Meaning	Example
0	No problem	No dependency or misuse of drugs
1	No/moderate problem due to help given	Receiving help for dependency or misuse
2	Serious problem	Dependency or misuse of prescribed, non-prescribed or illegal drugs
9	Not known	

If rated 0 or 9 go to next page

How much help with drug misuse does the person receive from friends or relatives?

Rating	Meaning	Example
0	None	
1	Low help	Occasional advice or support
2	Moderate help	Regular advice, put in touch with helping agencies
3	High help	Supervision, liaison with other agencies
9	Not known	

How much help with drug misuse does the person *receive* from local services?

How much help with drug misuse does the person *need* from local services for their drug misuse?

Rating	Meaning	Example
0	None	
1	Low help	Advice from GP
2	Moderate help	Drug dependency clinic
3	High help	Supervised withdrawal programme, in-patient care
9	Not known	

User's view of services required

Action(s)	By whom	Review date

14 Company

Are you happy with your social life?
Do you wish you had more contact with others?

Does the person need help with social contact?

Rating	Meaning	Example
0	No problem	Able to organise enough social contact, has enough friends
1	No/moderate problem due to help given	Attends appropriate drop-in or day centre
2	Serious problem	Frequently feels lonely and isolated
9	Not known	

If rated 0 or 9 go to next page

How much help with social contact does the person receive from friends or relatives?

Rating	Meaning	Example
0	None	
1	Low help	Social contact less than weekly
2	Moderate help	Social contact weekly or more often
3	High help	Social contact at least four times a week
9	Not known	

How much help does the person *receive* from local services in organising social contact?

How much help does the person *need* from local services in organising social contact?

Rating	Meaning	Example
0	None	
1	Low help	Given advice about social clubs
2	Moderate help	Day centre or community group up to 3 times a week
3	High help	Attends day centre 4 or more times a week
9	Not known	

User's view of services required

Action(s)

	By whom	Review date

15 Intimate relationships

Do you have a partner?
Do you have problems in your partnership/marriage?

Assessments

User rating · Staff rating

Does the person have any difficulty in finding a partner or in maintaining a close relationship?

Rating	Meaning	Example
0	No problem	Satisfactory relationship or happy not having partner
1	No/moderate problem due to help given	Receiving couple therapy, which is helpful
2	Serious problem	Domestic violence, wants partner
9	Not known	

If rated 0 or 9 go to next page

How much help with forming and maintaining close relationships does the person receive from friends or relatives?

Rating	Meaning	Example
0	None	
1	Low help	Some emotional support
2	Moderate help	Several talks, regular support
3	High help	Intensive talks and support in coping with feelings
9	Not known	

How much help with forming and maintaining close relationships does the person *receive* from local services?

How much help with forming and maintaining close relationships does the person *need* from local services?

Rating	Meaning	Example
0	None	
1	Low help	A few talks
2	Moderate help	Several talks, regular therapy
3	High help	Couple therapy, social skills training
9	Not known	

User's view of services required

Action(s)

	By whom	Review date

16 Sexual expression

How is your sex life?

Does the person have problems with his or her sex life?

Rating	Meaning	Example
0	No problem	Happy with current sex life
1	No/moderate problem due to help given	Benefiting from sexual therapy
2	Serious problem	Serious sexual difficulty, such as impotence
9	Not known	

If rated 0 or 9 go to next page

How much help with problems in his or her sex life does the person receive from friends or relatives?

Rating	Meaning	Example
0	None	
1	Low help	Some advice
2	Moderate help	Several talks, information material, providing contraceptives, etc
3	High help	Establish contact with counselling centres and possibly accompanying the person in going there. Consistent accessibility to talk about the problem.
9	Not known	

How much help with problems in his or her sex life does the person *receive* from local services?

How much help with problems in his or her sex life does the person *need* from local services?

Rating	Meaning	Example
0	None	
1	Low help	Given information about contraception, safe sex, drug-induced impotence
2	Moderate help	Regular talks about sex
3	High help	Sexual therapy
9	Not known	

User's view of services required

Action(s)

By whom	Review date

17 Child care

Do you have any children under 18?
Do you have any difficulty in looking after them?

Assessments

User rating   Staff rating

Does the person have difficulty looking after his or her children?

Rating	Meaning	Example
0	No problem	No children under 18 or no problem with looking after them
1	No/moderate problem due to help given	Difficulties with parenting and receiving help
2	Serious problem	Serious difficulty looking after children
9	Not known	

If rated 0 or 9 go to next page

How much help with looking after the children does the person receive from friends or relatives?

Rating	Meaning	Example
0	None	
1	Low help	Occasional babysitting less than once a week
2	Moderate help	Help most days
3	High help	Children living with friends or relatives
9	Not known	

How much help with looking after the children does the person *receive* from local services?

How much help with looking after the children does the person *need* from local services?

Rating	Meaning	Example
0	None	
1	Low help	Attending day nursery
2	Moderate help	Help with parenting skills
3	High help	Children in foster home, or in care
9	Not known	

User's view of services required

Action(s)	By whom	Review date

18 Basic education

Do you have difficulty in reading, writing or understanding English?
Can you count your change in a shop?

Does the person lack basic skills in numeracy and literacy?

Rating	Meaning	Example
0	No problem	Able to read, write and understand English forms
1	No/moderate problem due to help given	Difficulty with reading and has help from relative
2	Serious problem	Difficulty with basic skills, lack of English fluency
9	Not known	

If rated 0 or 9 go to next page

How much help with numeracy and literacy does the person receive from friends or relatives?

Rating	Meaning	Example
0	None	
1	Low help	Occasional help to read or write forms
2	Moderate help	Has put them in touch with literacy classes
3	High help	Teaches the person to read
9	Not known	

How much help with numeracy and literacy does the person *receive* from local services?

How much help with numeracy and literacy does the person *need* from local services?

Rating	Meaning	Example
0	None	
1	Low help	Help filling in forms
2	Moderate help	Given advice about classes
3	High help	Attending adult education
9	Not known	

User's view of services required

Action(s)	By whom	Review date

19 Telephone

Do you know how to use a telephone?
Is it easy to find one that you can use?

Does the person have any difficulty in getting access to or using a telephone?

Rating	Meaning	Example
0	No problem	Has working telephone in house or easy access to payphone
1	No/moderate problem due to help given	Has to request use of telephone
2	Serious problem	No access to telephone or unable to use telephone
9	Not known	

If rated 0 or 9 go to next page

How much help does the person receive from friends or relatives to make telephone calls?

Rating	Meaning	Example
0	None	
1	Low help	Help to make telephone calls but less than monthly or only for emergencies
2	Moderate help	Between monthly and daily
3	High help	Help available whenever wanted
9	Not known	

How much help does the person *receive* from local services to make telephone calls?

How much help does the person *need* from local services to make telephone calls?

Rating	Meaning	Example
0	None	
1	Low help	Access to telephone upon request
2	Moderate help	Provided with phonecard
3	High help	Arranges to have telephone fitted in home
9	Not known	

User's view of services required

Action(s)

	By whom	Review date

20 Transport

How do you find using the bus, tube or train?
Do you get a free bus pass?

Does the person have any problems using public transport?

Rating	Meaning	Example
0	No problem	Able to use public transport, or has access to car
1	No/moderate problem due to help given	Bus pass or other help provided with transport
2	Serious problem	Unable to use public transport
9	Not known	

If rated 0 or 9 go to next page

How much help with travelling does the person receive from friends or relatives?

Rating	Meaning	Example
0	None	
1	Low help	Encouragement to travel
2	Moderate help	Often accompanies on public transport
3	High help	Provides transport to all appointments
9	Not known	

How much help with travelling does the person *receive* from local services?

How much help with travelling does the person *need* from local services with travelling?

Rating	Meaning	Example
0	None	
1	Low help	Provision of bus pass
2	Moderate help	Taxi card
3	High help	Transport to appointments by ambulance
9	Not known	

User's view of services required

Action(s) | By whom | Review date

21 Money

How do you find budgeting your money?
Do you manage to pay your bills?

Does the person have problems budgeting his or her money?

Rating	Meaning	Example
0	No problem	Able to buy essential items and pay bills
1	No/moderate problem due to help given	Benefits from help with budgeting
2	Serious problem	Often has no money for essential items or bills
9	Not known	

If rated 0 or 9 go to next page

How much help does the person receive from friends or relatives in managing his or her money?

Rating	Meaning	Example
0	None	
1	Low help	Occasional help sorting out household bills
2	Moderate help	Calculating weekly budget
3	High help	Complete control of finance
9	Not known	

How much help does the person *receive* from local services in managing his or her money?

How much help does the person *need* from local services in managing his or her money?

Rating	Meaning	Example
0	None	
1	Low help	Occasional help with budgeting
2	Moderate help	Supervised in paying rent, given weekly spending money
3	High help	Daily handouts of cash
9	Not known	

User's view of services required

Action(s)	By whom	Review date

22 Benefits

Are you sure that you are getting all the money you are entitled to?

	User rating	Staff rating

Is the person definitely receiving all the benefits that he or she is entitled to?

Rating	Meaning	Example
0	No problem	Receiving full entitlement of benefits
1	No/moderate problem due to help given	Receives appropriate help in claiming benefits
2	Serious problem	Not sure/not receiving full entitlement of benefits
9	Not known	

If rated 0 or 9 then assessment is complete

How much help does the person receive from friends or relatives in obtaining the full benefit entitlement?

Rating	Meaning	Example
0	None	
1	Low help	Occasionally asks whether person is getting any money
2	Moderate help	Has helped fill in forms
3	High help	Has made enquiries about full entitlement
9	Not known	

How much help does the person *receive* from local services in obtaining the full benefit entitlement?

How much help does the person *need* from local services in obtaining the full benefit entitlement?

Rating	Meaning	Example
0	None	
1	Low help	Occasional advice about entitlements
2	Moderate help	Help with applying for extra entitlements
3	High help	Comprehensive evaluation of current entitlement
9	Not known	

User's view of services required

Action(s)

	By whom	Review date

Appendix 3

CAN–C Summary scoring sheets

CAN–C
Complete assessment summary sheet

User name _____   Date of assessment ____/____/____

Staff name _____   Date of assessment ____/____/____

	Need		Informal help given		Formal help given		Formal help needed		User's views recorded?	Action plan?
Rating	0,1,2,9		0,1,2,3,9		0,1,2,3,9		0,1,2,3,9		Yes	Review date
User/Staff rating	U	S	U	S	U	S	U	S	U	S
1 Accommodation										
2 Food										
3 Looking after home										
4 Self-care										
5 Daytime activities										
6 Physical health										
7 Psychotic symptoms										
8 Information										
9 Psychological distress										
10 Safety to self										
11 Safety to others										
12 Alcohol										
13 Drugs										
14 Company										
15 Intimate relationships										
16 Sexual expression										
17 Child care										
18 Education										
19 Telephone										
20 Transport										
21 Money										
22 Benefits										
Number of met needs (Number of 1s)										
Number of unmet needs (Number of 2s)										
Total number of needs (Number of 1s and 2s)										
Total level of help given & needed (Add scores, rate 9 as 0)										

CAN–C
User assessment summary sheet

User name _____   Date of assessment _____/_____/_____

Interviewer _____

	Need	Informal help given	Formal help given	Formal help needed	User's views recorded?	Action plan?
Rating	0,1,2,9	0,1,2,3,9	0,1,2,3,9	0,1,2,3,9	Yes	Review date
1 Accommodation						
2 Food						
3 Looking after home						
4 Self-care						
5 Daytime activities						
6 Physical health						
7 Psychotic symptoms						
8 Information						
9 Psychological distress						
10 Safety to self						
11 Safety to others						
12 Alcohol						
13 Drugs						
14 Company						
15 Intimate relationships						
16 Sexual expression						
17 Child care						
18 Education						
19 Telephone						
20 Transport						
21 Money						
22 Benefits						
Number of met needs (Number of 1s)						
Number of unmet needs (Number of 2s)						
Total number of needs (Number of 1s and 2s)						
Total level of help given & needed (Add scores, rate 9 as 0)						

CAN-C
Staff assessment summary sheet

User name _____

Staff name _____   Date of assessment _____/_____/_____

	Need	Informal help given	Formal help given	Formal help needed	Action plan?
Rating	0,1,2,9	0,1,2,3,9	0,1,2,3,9	0,1,2,3,9	Review date
1 Accommodation					
2 Food					
3 Looking after home					
4 Self-care					
5 Daytime activities					
6 Physical health					
7 Psychotic symptoms					
8 Information					
9 Psychological distress					
10 Safety to self					
11 Safety to others					
12 Alcohol					
13 Drugs					
14 Company					
15 Intimate relationships					
16 Sexual expression					
17 Child care					
18 Education					
19 Telephone					
20 Transport					
21 Money					
22 Benefits					
Number of met needs (Number of 1s)					
Number of unmet needs (Number of 2s)					
Total number of needs (Number of 1s and 2s)					
Total level of help given & needed (Add scores, rate 9 as 0)					

Appendix 4

Camberwell Assessment of Need – Research version (CAN–R)

How to use the CAN–R

What is the CAN–R?

The CAN–R is a tool for the comprehensive assessment of the needs of people with severe mental health problems. It is designed for research use, in conjunction with Chapter 6. Interviewers will need to have experience of clinical assessment interviews, and reliability will be increased by using the training programme contained in Chapter 7.

How do I complete the CAN–R?

The CAN–R assesses problems during the last one month in 22 domains of life. This relatively short time span leads to a snapshot of the current situation. Assessment involves separate interviews with the user (the term used to cover patient/client/consumer – the person being assessed) and a staff member who knows the service user sufficiently well. It is important that the interviewee's response is recorded directly even if the interviewer disagrees with this view – user and staff perceptions of need do differ.

Each page contains four sections (each in a box). Use the suggested questions above Section 1 (shown in italics) to open discussion on each domain. Supplementary questions should be asked where necessary, with the goal of establishing:

(a)   whether the user has a serious problem in this doamin; and
(b)   if the user does have a serious problem, whether he or she is getting effective help.

On the basis of the interviewee's responses, a *need rating* is made for the last month:

0 = no serious problem (i.e. no need)
1 = no/moderate problem due to help given (i.e. met need)
2 = serious problem (i.e. unmet need, whether or not help is given)
9 = not known

The need rating is made using the following guidelines:

- If a serious problem is present (regardless of cause, and whether or not any help is being given), then **rate 2**.
- If there is *no* serious problem *because* help is being given (e.g. family support, sheltered housing, psychotherapy, medication), then **rate 1**.
- If there are no problems in this area, then **rate 0**.
- If the person being interviewed does not know or does not want to answer questions on this domain, then **rate 9**.

If a need is not identified, then go on to the next domain. Sections 2–4 are only completed if a need is identified (i.e. need rating is 1 or 2). Section 2 assesses help received from informal sources (e.g.

friends, family, neighbours) and Section 3 the help received from formal sources (e.g. health, housing and social services). Section 3 also records the interviewee's perceptions of help needed, to allow undermet need to be identified. Section 4 records satisfaction with current help. Note that only the user is asked if they are satisfied with the amount of help.

Note

- Just because there is currently no problem, the need rating is not automatically 0. For example a person with diabetes who is well because of the prescribed insulin would be rated as 1 for physical health.
- A need can exist for a variety of reasons. For example, a person with a psychotic illness may currently be unable to go shopping because of a sprained ankle. He or she should be rated as having a need (i.e. need rating 1 or 2) in the Food domain, even though this need is not related to his or her psychiatric condition.
- The CAN–R does not assess over-provision of services. For example, if a person was an in-patient for the last month, but has what he or she considers consider to be adequate accommodation outside hospital, then accommodation should be rated as 0, even though he or she is currently being provided with hospital accommodation.

Contents

1   Accommodation

What kind of place do you live in?
What sort of place is it?

Assessments

User rating   Staff rating

Does the person lack a current place to stay?

CAN011U   CAN011S

Rating	Meaning	Example
0	No problem	Person does have an adequate home (even if in hospital currently)
1	No/moderate problem due to help given	Person is living in sheltered accommodation or hostel
2	Serious problem	Person is homeless, precariously housed, or home lacks basic facilities such as water and electricity
9	Not known	

If rated 0 or 9 go to next page

How much help with accommodation does the person receive from friends or relatives?

CAN012U   CAN012S

Rating	Meaning	Example
0	None	
1	Low help	Occasionally supplied with a few pieces of furniture
2	Moderate help	Substantial help with improving accommodation, such as redecoration of flat
3	High help	Living with relative because own accommodation is unsatisfactory
9	Not known	

How much help with accommodation does the person *receive* from local services?

CAN013U   CAN013S

How much help with accommodation does the person *need* from local services?

CAN014U   CAN014S

Rating	Meaning	Example
0	None	
1	Low help	Minor decoration, address of housing agency
2	Moderate help	Major improvements, referral to housing agency
3	High help	Being rehoused, living in group home or hostel
9	Not known	

Does the person receive the right type of help with accommodation?

CAN015U   CAN015S

(0=No; 1=Yes; 9=Not known)

Overall, is the person satisfied with the amount of help he or she is receiving with accommodation?

CAN016U

(0=Not satisfied; 1=Satisfied; 9=Not known)

2 Food

What kind of food do you eat?
Are you able to prepare your own meals and do your own shopping?

Does the person have difficulty in getting enough to eat?

CAN021U   CAN021S

Rating	Meaning	Example
0	No problem	Able to buy and prepare meals
1	No/moderate problem due to help given	Unable to prepare food and has meals provided
2	Serious problem	Very restricted diet, culturally inappropriate food
9	Not known	

If rated 0 or 9 go to next page

How much help with getting enough to eat does the person receive from friends or relatives?

CAN022U   CAN022S

Rating	Meaning	Example
0	None	
1	Low help	Meal provided weekly or less
2	Moderate help	Weekly help with shopping or meals provided more than weekly but not daily
3	High help	Meal provided daily
9	Not known	

How much help with getting enough to eat does the person *receive* from local services?

CAN023U   CAN023S

How much help with getting enough to eat does the person *need* from local services?

CAN024U   CAN024S

Rating	Meaning	Example
0	None	
1	Low help	1–4 meals a week provided, or assisted for one meal a day
2	Moderate help	More than 4 meals a week provided, or assisted for all meals
3	High help	All meals provided
9	Not known	

Does the person receive the right type of help with getting enough to eat?

CAN025U   CAN025S

(0=No; 1=Yes; 9=Not known)

Overall, is the person satisfied with the amount of help he or she is receiving in getting enough to eat?

CAN026U

(0=Not satisfied; 1=Satisfied; 9=Not known)

---

3 Looking after the home

Are you able to look after your home?
Does anyone help you?

Assessments

User rating | Staff rating

Does the person have difficulty looking after the home?

CAN031U   CAN031S

Rating	Meaning	Example
0	No problem	Home may be untidy but the person keeps it basically clean
1	No/moderate problem due to help given	Unable to look after home and has regular domestic help
2	Serious problem	Home is dirty and a potential health hazard
9	Not known	

If rated 0 or 9 go to next page

How much help with looking after the home does the person receive from friends or relatives?

CAN032U   CAN032S

Rating	Meaning	Example
0	None	
1	Low help	Prompts or helps tidy up or clean occasionally
2	Moderate help	Prompts or helps clean at least once a week
3	High help	Supervises the person more than once a week, washes all clothes and cleans the home
9	Not known	

How much help does the person *receive* from local services with looking after the home?

CAN033U   CAN033S

How much help does the person *need* from local services with looking after their home?

CAN034U   CAN034S

Rating	Meaning	Example
0	None	
1	Low help	Prompting by staff
2	Moderate help	Some assistance with household tasks
3	High help	Majority of household tasks done by staff
9	Not known	

Does the person receive the right type of help with looking after the home?

CAN035U   CAN035S

(0=No; 1=Yes; 9=Not known)

Overall, is the person satisfied with the amount of help he or she is receiving in looking after the home?

CAN036U

(0=Not satisfied; 1=Satisfied; 9=Not known)

4 Self-care

Do you have problems keeping clean and tidy?
Do you ever need reminding? Who by?

Does the person have difficulty with self-care?

CAN041U   CAN041S

Rating	Meaning	Example
0	No problem	Appearance may be eccentric or untidy, but basically clean
1	No/moderate problem due to help given	Needs and gets help with self-care
2	Serious problem	Poor personal hygiene, smells
9	Not known	

If rated 0 or 9 go to next page

How much help does the person receive from friends or relatives with their self-care?

CAN042U   CAN042S

Rating	Meaning	Example
0	None	
1	Low help	Occasionally prompt the person to change their clothes
2	Moderate help	Run the bath/shower and insist on its use, daily prompting
3	High help	Provide daily assistance with several aspects of care
9	Not known	

How much help does the person *receive* from local services with their self-care?

CAN043U   CAN043S

How much help does the person *need* from local services with their self-care?

CAN044U   CAN044S

Rating	Meaning	Example
0	None	
1	Low help	Occasional prompting
2	Moderate help	Supervise weekly washing
3	High help	Supervise several aspects of self-care, self-care skills programme
9	Not known	

Does the person receive the right type of help with self-care?

CAN045U   CAN045S

(0=No; 1=Yes; 9=Not known)

Overall, is the person satisfied with the amount of help they are receiving with self-care?

CAN046U

(0=Not satisfied; 1=Satisfied; 9=Not known)

5   Daytime activities

How do you spend your day?
Do you have enough to do?

Assessments

	User rating	Staff rating

Does the person have difficulty with regular, appropriate daytime activities?

CAN051U   CAN051S

Rating	Meaning	Example
0	No problem	In full time employment, or adequately occupied with household/social activities
1	No/moderate problem due to help given	Unable to occupy self, so attending day centre
2	Serious problem	No employment of any kind and not adequately occupied with household/social activities
9	Not known	

If rated 0 or 9 go to next page

How much help does the person receive from friends or relatives in finding or keeping regular, appropriate daytime activities?

CAN052U   CAN052S

Rating	Meaning	Example
0	None	
1	Low help	Occasional advice about daytime activities
2	Moderate help	Has arranged daytime activities such as adult education or day centre attendance
3	High help	Daily help with arranging daytime activities
9	Not known	

How much help does the person *receive* from local services in finding or keeping regular, appropriate daytime activities?

CAN053U   CAN053S

How much help does the person *need* from local services in finding or keeping regular, appropriate daytime activities?

CAN054U   CAN054S

Rating	Meaning	Example
0	None	
1	Low help	Employment training / adult education
2	Moderate help	Sheltered employment daily. Day centre 2–4 days a week
3	High help	Attends day hospital or day centre daily
9	Not known	

Does the person receive the right type of help with getting daytime activities?

CAN055U   CAN055S

(0=No; 1=Yes; 9=Not known)

Overall, is the person satisfied with the amount of help he or she is receiving with daytime activities?

CAN056U

(0=Not satisfied; 1=Satisfied; 9=Not known)

6   Physical health

How well do you feel physically?
Are you getting any treatment for physical problems from your doctor?

Assessments

User rating	Staff rating

Does the person have any physical disability or any physical illness?

CAN061U   CAN061S

Rating	Meaning	Example
0	No problem	Physically well
1	No/moderate problem due to help given	Physical ailment, such as high blood pressure, receiving appropriate treatment
2	Serious problem	Untreated physical ailment, including side-effects
9	Not known	

If rated 0 or 9 go to next page

How much help does the person receive from friends or relatives for physical health problems?

CAN062U   CAN062S

Rating	Meaning	Example
0	None	
1	Low help	Prompting to go to doctor
2	Moderate help	Accompanied to doctor
3	High help	Daily help with going to the toilet, eating or mobility
9	Not known	

How much help does the person *receive* from local services for physical health problems?

CAN063U   CAN063S

How much help does the person *need* from local services for physical health problems?

CAN064U   CAN064S

Rating	Meaning	Example
0	None	
1	Low help	Given dietary or family planning advice
2	Moderate help	Prescribed medication. Regularly seen by GP/nurse
3	High help	Frequent hospital appointments. Alterations to home
9	Not known	

Does the person receive the right type of help for physical problems?

CAN065U   CAN065S

(0=No; 1=Yes; 9=Not known)

Overall, is the person satisfied with the amount of help he or she is receiving for physical problems?

CAN066U

(0=Not satisfied; 1=Satisfied; 9=Not known)

7 Psychotic symptoms

Do you ever hear voices, or have problems with your thoughts?
Are you on any medication or injections? What is it for?

Assessments

| User rating | Staff rating |

Does the person have any psychotic symptoms?

CAN071U CAN071S

Rating	Meaning	Example
0	No problem	No positive symptoms, not at risk from symptoms and not on medication
1	No/moderate problem due to help given	Symptoms helped by medication or other help
2	Serious problem	Currently has symptoms or at risk
9	Not known	

If rated 0 or 9 go to next page

How much help does the person receive from friends or relatives for these psychotic symptoms?

CAN072U CAN072S

Rating	Meaning	Example
0	None	
1	Low help	Some sympathy and support
2	Moderate help	Carers involved in helping with coping strategies or medication compliance
3	High help	Constant supervision of medication, and help with coping strategies
9	Not known	

How much help does the person *receive* from local services for these psychotic symptoms?

CAN073U CAN073S

How much help does the person *need* from local services for these psychotic symptoms?

CAN074U CAN074S

Rating	Meaning	Example
0	None	
1	Low help	Medication reviewed thrice monthly or less, support group
2	Moderate help	Medication reviewed more than thrice monthly, structured psychological therapy
3	High help	Medication and 24-hour hospital care or crisis care at home
9	Not known	

Does the person receive the right type of help for psychotic symptoms?

CAN075U CAN075S

(0=No; 1=Yes; 9=Not known)

Overall, is the person satisfied with the amount of help he or she is receiving for psychotic symptoms?

CAN076U

(0=Not satisfied; 1=Satisfied; 9=Not known)

8 Information on condition and treatment

Have you been given clear information about your medication or other treatment?
How helpful has the information been?

Assessments

User rating   Staff rating

Has the person had clear verbal or written information about condition and treatment?

CAN081U   CAN081S

Rating	Meaning	Example
0	No problem	Has received and understood adequate information
1	No/moderate problem due to help given	Has not received or understood all information
2	Serious problem	Has received no information
9	Not known	

If rated 0 or 9 go to next page

How much help does the person receive from friends or relatives in obtaining such information?

CAN082U   CAN082S

Rating	Meaning	Example
0	None	
1	Low help	Has had some advice from friends or relatives
2	Moderate help	Given leaflets/factsheets or put in touch with self-help groups by friends or relatives
3	High help	Regular liaison with doctors or groups such as MIND, by friends or relatives
9	Not known	

How much help does the person *receive* from local services in obtaining such information?

CAN083U   CAN083S

How much help does the person *need* from local services in obtaining such information?

CAN084U   CAN084S

Rating	Meaning	Example
0	None	
1	Low help	Brief verbal or written information on illness/problem/treatment
2	Moderate help	Given details of self-help groups. Long verbal information sessions on drugs and alternative treatments.
3	High help	Has been given detailed written information or has had specific personal education
9	Not known	

Does the person receive the right type of help in obtaining information?

CAN085U   CAN085S

(0=No; 1=Yes; 9=Not known)

Overall, is the person satisfied with the amount of help he or she is receiving in obtaining information?

CAN086U

(0=Not satisfied; 1=Satisfied; 9=Not known)

9   Psychological distress

Have you recently felt very sad or low?
Have you felt overly anxious or frightened?

Does the person suffer from current psychological distress?

CAN091U   CAN091S

Rating	Meaning	Example
0	No problem	Occasional or mild distress
1	No/moderate problem due to help given	Needs and gets ongoing support
2	Serious problem	Has expressed suicidal ideas during last month or has exposed themselves to serious danger
9	Not known	

If rated 0 or 9 go to next page

How much help does the person receive from friends or relatives for this distress?

CAN092U   CAN092S

Rating	Meaning	Example
0	None	
1	Low help	Some sympathy or support
2	Moderate help	Has opportunity at least weekly to talk about distress to friend or relative
3	High help	Constant support and supervision
9	Not known	

How much help does the person *receive* from local services for this distress?

CAN093U   CAN093S

How much help does the person *need* from local services for this distress?

CAN094U   CAN094S

Rating	Meaning	Example
0	None	
1	Low help	Assessment of mental state or occasional support
2	Moderate help	Specific psychological or social treatment for anxiety. Counselled by staff at least once a week
3	High help	24-hour hospital care or crisis care
9	Not known	

Does the person receive the right type of help for this distress?

CAN095U   CAN095S

(0=No; 1=Yes; 9=Not known)

Overall, is the person satisfied with the amount of help he or she is receiving for this distress?

CAN096U

(0=Not satisfied; 1=Satisfied; 9=Not known)

10 Safety to self

Do you ever have thoughts of harming yourself, or actually harm yourself?
Do you put yourself in danger in other ways?

Assessments

User rating | Staff rating

Is the person a danger to him- or herself?

CAN101U   CAN101S

Rating	Meaning	Example
0	No problem	No suicidal thoughts
1	No/moderate problem due to help given	Suicide risk monitored by staff, receiving counselling
2	Serious problem	Distress affects life significantly, such as preventing person going out
9	Not known	

If rated 0 or 9 go to next page

How much help does the person receive from friends or relatives to reduce the risk of self-harm?

CAN102U   CAN102S

Rating	Meaning	Example
0	None	
1	Low help	Able to contact friends or relatives if feeling unsafe
2	Moderate help	Friends or relatives are usually in contact and are likely to know if feeling unsafe
3	High help	Friends or relatives in regular contact and are very likely to know and provide help if feeling unsafe
9	Not known	

How much help does the person *receive* from local services to reduce the risk of self-harm?

CAN103U   CAN103S

How much help does the person *need* from local services to reduce the risk of self-harm?

CAN104U   CAN104S

Rating	Meaning	Example
0	None	
1	Low help	Someone to contact when feeling unsafe
2	Moderate help	Staff check at least once a week, regular supportive counselling
3	High help	Daily supervision, in-patient care
9	Not known	

Does the person receive the right type of help to reduce the risk of self-harm?

CAN105U   CAN105S

(0=No; 1=Yes; 9=Not known)

Overall, is the person satisfied with the amount of help they are receiving to reduce the risk of self-harm?

CAN106U

(0=Not satisfied; 1=Satisfied; 9=Not known)

11 Safety to others

Do you think you could be a danger to other people's safety?
Do you ever lose your temper and hit someone?

Assessments

User rating | Staff rating

Is the person a current or potential risk to other people's safety?

CAN111U CAN111S

Rating	Meaning	Example
0	No problem	No history of violence or threatening behaviour
1	No/moderate problem due to help given	At risk from alcohol misuse and receiving help
2	Serious problem	Recent violence or threats
9	Not known	

If rated 0 or 9 go to next page

How much help does the person receive from friends or relatives to reduce the risk that he or she might harm someone else?

CAN112U CAN112S

Rating	Meaning	Example
0	None	
1	Low help	Help with threatening behaviour weekly or less
2	Moderate help	Help with threatening behaviour more than weekly
3	High help	Almost constant help with persistently threatening behaviour
9	Not known	

How much help does the person *receive* from local services to reduce the risk that he or she might harm someone else?

CAN113U CAN113S

How much help does the person *need* from local services to reduce the risk that he or she might harm someone else?

CAN114U CAN114S

Rating	Meaning	Example
0	None	
1	Low help	Check on behaviour weekly or less
2	Moderate help	Daily supervision
3	High help	Constant supervision. Anger management programme
9	Not know	

Does the person receive the right type of help to reduce the risk that he or she might harm someone else?

CAN115U CAN115S

(0=No; 1=Yes; 9=Not known)

Overall, is the person satisfied with the amount of help they are receiving to reduce the risk that he or she might harm someone else?

CAN116U

(0=Not satisfied; 1=Satisfied; 9=Not known)

12 Alcohol

Does drinking cause you any problems?
Do you wish you could cut down your drinking?

User rating   Staff rating

Does the person drink excessively, or have a problem controlling his or her drinking?

CAN121U   CAN121S

Rating	Meaning	Example
0	No problem	No problem with controlled drinking
1	No/moderate problem due to help given	Under supervision because of potential risk
2	Serious problem	Current drinking harmful or uncontrollable
9	Not known	

If rated 0 or 9 go to next page

How much help does the person receive from friends or relatives for their drinking?

CAN122U   CAN122S

Rating	Meaning	Example
0	None	
1	Low help	Told to cut down
2	Moderate help	Advised about Alcoholics Anonymous
3	High help	Daily monitoring of alcohol
9	Not known	

How much help does the person *receive* from local services for this drinking?

CAN123U   CAN123S

How much help does the person *need* from local services for this drinking?

CAN124U   CAN124S

Rating	Meaning	Example
0	None	
1	Low help	Told about risks
2	Moderate help	Given details of helping agencies
3	High help	Attends alcohol clinic, supervised withdrawal programme
9	Not known	

Does the person receive the right type of help for this drinking?

CAN125U   CAN125S

(0=No; 1=Yes; 9=Not known)

Overall, is the person satisfied with the amount of help he or she is receiving for this drinking?

CAN126U

(0=Not satisfied; 1=Satisfied; 9=Not known)

13 Drugs

Do you take any drugs that aren't prescribed?
Are there any drugs you would find hard to stop taking?

Assessments

User rating	Staff rating

Does the person have problems with drug misuse?

CAN131U   CAN131S

Rating	Meaning	Example
0	No problem	No dependency or misuse of drugs
1	No/moderate problem due to help given	Receiving help for dependency or misuse
2	Serious problem	Dependency or misuse of prescribed, non-prescribed or illegal drugs
9	Not known	

If rated 0 or 9 go to next page

How much help with drug misuse does the person receive from friends or relatives?

CAN132U   CAN132S

Rating	Meaning	Example
0	None	
1	Low help	Occasional advice or support
2	Moderate help	Regular advice, put in touch with helping agencies
3	High help	Supervision, liaison with other agencies
9	Not known	

How much help with drug misuse does the person *receive* from local services?

CAN133U   CAN133S

How much help with drug misuse does the person *need* from local services?

CAN134U   CAN134S

Rating	Meaning	Example
0	None	
1	Low help	Advice from GP
2	Moderate help	Drug dependency clinic
3	High help	Supervised withdrawal programme, in-patient care
9	Not known	

Does the person receive the right type of help for drug misuse?

CAN135U   CAN135S

(0=No; 1=Yes; 9=Not known)

Overall, is the person satisfied with the amount of help he or she is receiving for drug misuse?

CAN136U

(0=Not satisfied; 1=Satisfied; 9=Not known)

14 Company

Are you happy with your social life?
Do you wish you had more contact with others?

Assessments

User rating · Staff rating

Does the person need help with social contact?

CAN141U · CAN141S

Rating	Meaning	Example
0	No problem	Able to organise enough social contact, has enough friends
1	No/moderate problem due to help given	Attends appropriate drop-in or day centre
2	Serious problem	Frequently feels lonely and isolated
9	Not known	

If rated 0 or 9 go to next page

How much help with social contact does the person receive from friends or relatives?

CAN142U · CAN142S

Rating	Meaning	Example
0	None	
1	Low help	Social contact less than weekly
2	Moderate help	Social contact weekly or more often
3	High help	Social contact at least four times a week
9	Not known	

How much help does the person *receive* from local services in organising social contact?

CAN143U · CAN143S

How much help does the person *need* from local services in organising social contact?

CAN144U · CAN144S

Rating	Meaning	Example
0	None	
1	Low help	Given advice about social clubs
2	Moderate help	Day centre or community group up to 3 times a week
3	High help	Attends day centre 4 or more times a week
9	Not known	

Does the person receive the right type of help in organising social contact?

CAN145U · CAN145S

(0=No; 1=Yes; 9=Not known)

Overall, is the person satisfied with the amount of help he or she is receiving in organising social contact?

CAN146U

(0=Not satisfied; 1=Satisfied; 9=Not known)

15 Intimate relationships

Do you have a partner?
Do you have problems in your partnership/marriage?

Does the person have any difficulty in finding a partner or in maintaining a close relationship?

CAN151U · CAN151S

Rating	Meaning	Example
0	No problem	Satisfactory relationship or happy not having partner
1	No/moderate problem due to help given	Receiving couple therapy, which is helpful
2	Serious problem	Domestic violence, wants partner
9	Not known	

If rated 0 or 9 go to next page

How much help does the person receive from friends or relatives with forming and maintaining close relationships?

CAN152U · CAN152S

Rating	Meaning	Example
0	None	
1	Low help	Some emotional support
2	Moderate help	Several talks, regular support
3	High help	Intensive talks and support in coping with feelings
9	Not known	

How much help does the person *receive* from local services with forming and maintaining close relationships?

CAN153U · CAN153S

How much help does the person *need* from local services with forming and maintaining close relationships?

CAN154U · CAN154S

Rating	Meaning	Example
0	None	
1	Low help	A few talks
2	Moderate help	Several talks, regular therapy
3	High help	Couple therapy, social skills training
9	Not known	

Does the person receive the right type of help with forming and maintaining close relationships?

CAN155U · CAN155S

(0=No; 1=Yes; 9=Not known)

Overall, is the person satisfied with the amount of help he or she is receiving with forming and maintaining close relationships?

CAN156U

(0=Not satisfied; 1=Satisfied; 9=Not known)

16 Sexual expression

How is your sex life?

Does the person have problems with his or her sex life?

CAN161U   CAN161S

Rating	Meaning	Example
0	No problem	Happy with current sex life
1	No/moderate problem due to help given	Benefiting from sexual therapy
2	Serious problem	Serious sexual difficulty, such as impotence
9	Not known	

If rated 0 or 9 go to next page

How much help with problems in his or her does the person receive from friends or relatives sex life?

CAN162U   CAN162S

Rating	Meaning	Example
0	None	
1	Low help	Some advice
2	Moderate help	Several talks, information material, providing contraceptives, etc
3	High help	Establish contact with counselling centres and possibly accompanying the person in going there. Consistent accessibility to talk about the problem.
9	Not known	

How much help with problems in his or her sex life does the person *receive* from local services?

CAN163U   CAN163S

How much help with problems in his or her sex life does the person *need* from local services?

CAN164U   CAN164S

Rating	Meaning	Example
0	None	
1	Low help	Given information about contraception, safe sex, drug-induced impotence
2	Moderate help	Regular talks about sex
3	High help	Sexual therapy
9	Not known	

Does the person receive the right type of help for problems in his or her sex life?

CAN165U   CAN165S

(0=No; 1=Yes; 9=Not known)

Overall, is the person satisfied with the amount of help he or she is receiving for problems in his or her sex life?

CAN166U

(0=Not satisfied; 1=Satisfied; 9=Not known)

17 Child care

Do you have any children under 18?
Do you have any difficulty in looking after them?

Assessments

User rating | Staff rating

Does the person have difficulty looking after his or her children?

CAN171U   CAN171S

Rating	Meaning	Example
0	No problem	No children under 18 or no problem with looking after them
1	No/moderate problem due to help given	Difficulties with parenting and receiving help
2	Serious problem	Serious difficulty looking after children
9	Not known	

If rated 0 or 9 go to next page

How much help with looking after the children does the person receive from friends or relatives?

CAN172U   CAN172S

Rating	Meaning	Example
0	None	
1	Low help	Occasional babysitting less than once a week
2	Moderate help	Help most days
3	High help	Children living with friends or relatives
9	Not known	

How much help with looking after their children does the person *receive* from local services?

CAN173U   CAN173S

How much help with looking after their children does the person *need* from local services?

CAN174U   CAN174S

Rating	Meaning	Example
0	None	
1	Low help	Attending day nursery
2	Moderate help	Help with parenting skills
3	High help	Children in foster home, or in care
9	Not known	

Does the person receive the right type of help for looking after the children?

CAN175U   CAN175S

(0=No; 1=Yes; 9=Not known)

Overall, is the person satisfied with the amount of help he or she is receiving for looking after the children?

CAN176U

(0=Not satisfied; 1=Satisfied; 9=Not known)

18 Basic education

Do you have difficulty in reading, writing or understanding English?
Can you count your change in a shop?

Assessments

User rating   Staff rating

Does the person lack basic skills in numeracy and literacy?

CAN181U   CAN181S

Rating	Meaning	Example
0	No problem	Able to read, write and understand English forms
1	No/moderate problem due to help given	Difficulty with reading and has help from relatives
2	Serious problem	Difficulty with basic skills, lack of English fluency
9	Not known	

If rated 0 or 9 go to next page

How much help with numeracy and literacy does the person receive from friends or relatives?

CAN182U   CAN182S

Rating	Meaning	Example
0	None	
1	Low help	Occasional help to read or write forms
2	Moderate help	Has put them in touch with literacy classes
3	High help	Teaches the person to read
9	Not known	

How much help with numeracy and literacy does the person *receive* from local services?

CAN183U   CAN183S

How much help with numeracy and literacy does the person *need* from local services?

CAN184U   CAN184S

Rating	Meaning	Example
0	None	
1	Low help	Help filling in forms
2	Moderate help	Given advice about classes
3	High help	Attending adult education
9	Not known	

Does the person receive the right type of help with numeracy and literacy?

CAN185U   CAN185S

(0=No; 1=Yes; 9=Not known)

Overall, is the person satisfied with the amount of help he or she is receiving with numeracy and literacy?

CAN186U

(0=Not satisfied; 1=Satisfied; 9=Not known)

19 Telephone

Do you know how to use a telephone?
Is it easy to find one that you can use?

Assessments

| User rating | Staff rating |

Does the person have any difficulty in getting access to or using a telephone?

CAN191U   CAN191S

Rating	Meaning	Example
0	No problem	Has working telephone in house or easy access to payphone
1	No/moderate problem due to help given	Has to request use of telephone
2	Serious problem	No access to telephone or unable to use telephone
9	Not known	

If rated 0 or 9 go to next page

How much help does the person receive from friends or relatives to make telephone calls?

CAN192U   CAN192S

Rating	Meaning	Example
0	None	
1	Low help	Help to make telephone calls but less than monthly or only for emergencies
2	Moderate help	Between monthly and daily
3	High help	Help available whenever wanted
9	Not known	

How much help does the person *receive* from local services to make telephone calls?

CAN193U   CAN193S

How much help does the person *need* from local services to make telephone calls?

CAN194U   CAN194S

Rating	Meaning	Example
0	None	
1	Low help	Access to telephone upon request
2	Moderate help	Provided with phonecard
3	High help	Arranges to have telephone fitted in home
9	Not known	

Does the person receive the right type of help to make telephone calls?

CAN195U   CAN195S

(0=No; 1=Yes; 9=Not known)

Overall, is the person satisfied with the amount of help he or she is receiving to make telephone calls?

CAN196U

(0=Not satisfied; 1=Satisfied; 9=Not known)

20 Transport

How do you find using the bus, tube or train?
Do you get a free bus pass?

Does the person have any problems using public transport?

CAN201U   CAN201S

Rating	Meaning	Example
0	No problem	Able to use public transport, or has access to car
1	No/moderate problem due to help given	Bus pass or other help provided with transport
2	Serious problem	Unable to use public transport
9	Not known	

If rated 0 or 9 go to next page

How much help with travelling does the person receive from friends or relatives?

CAN202U   CAN202S

Rating	Meaning	Example
0	None	
1	Low help	Encouragement to travel
2	Moderate help	Often accompanies on public transport
3	High help	Provides transport to all appointments
9	Not known	

How much help does the person *receive* from local services with travelling?

CAN203U   CAN203S

How much help does the person *need* from local services with travelling?

CAN204U   CAN204S

Rating	Meaning	Example
0	None	
1	Low help	Provision of bus pass
2	Moderate help	Taxi card
3	High help	Transport to appointments by ambulance
9	Not known	

Does the person receive the right type of help with travelling?

CAN205U   CAN205S

(0=No; 1=Yes; 9=Not known)

Overall, is the person satisfied with the amount of help he or she is receiving with travelling?

CAN206U

(0=Not satisfied; 1=Satisfied; 9=Not known)

21 Money

How do you find budgeting your money?
Do you manage to pay your bills?

Does the person have problems budgeting his or her money?

CAN211U   CAN211S

Rating	Meaning	Example
0	No problem	Able to buy essential items and pay bills
1	No/moderate problem due to help given	Benefits from help with budgeting
2	Serious problem	Often has no money for essential items or bills
9	Not known	

If rated 0 or 9 go to next page

How much help does the person receive from friends or relatives in managing his or her money?

CAN212U   CAN212S

Rating	Meaning	Example
0	None	
1	Low help	Occasional help sorting out household bills
2	Moderate help	Calculating weekly budget
3	High help	Complete control of finance
9	Not known	

How much help does the person *receive* from local services in managing his or her money?

CAN213U   CAN213S

How much help does the person *need* from local services in managing his or her money?

CAN214U   CAN214S

Rating	Meaning	Example
0	None	
1	Low help	Occasional help with budgeting
2	Moderate help	Supervised in paying rent, given weekly spending money
3	High help	Daily handouts of cash
9	Not known	

Does the person receive the right type of help in managing his or her money?

CAN215U   CAN215S

(0=No; 1=Yes; 9=Not known)

Overall, is the person satisfied with the amount of help he or she is receiving in managing his or her money?

CAN216U

(0=Not satisfied; 1=Satisfied; 9=Not known)

22 Benefits

Are you sure that you are getting all the money you are entitled to?

Is the person definitely receiving all the benefits that he or she is entitled to?

CAN221U   CAN221S

Rating	Meaning	Example
0	No problem	Receiving full entitlement of benefits
1	No/moderate problem due to help given	Receives appropriate help in claiming benefits
2	Serious problem	Not sure/not receiving full entitlement of benefits
9	Not known	

If rated 0 or 9 the assessment is complete

How much help does the person receive from friends or relatives in obtaining the full benefit entitlement?

CAN222U   CAN222S

Rating	Meaning	Example
0	None	
1	Low help	Occasionally asks whether person is getting any money
2	Moderate help	Has helped fill in forms
3	High help	Has made enquiries about full entitlement
9	Not known	

How much help does the person *receive* from local services in obtaining the full benefit entitlement?

CAN223U   CAN223S

How much help does the person *need* from local services in obtaining the full benefit entitlement?

CAN224U   CAN224S

Rating	Meaning	Example
0	None	
1	Low help	Occasional advice about entitlements
2	Moderate help	Help with applying for extra entitlements
3	High help	Comprehensive evaluation of current entitlement
9	Not known	

Does the person receive the right type of help in obtaining the full benefit entitlement?

CAN225U   CAN225S

(0=No; 1=Yes; 9=Not known)

Overall, is the person satisfied with the amount of help he or she is receiveng in obtaining the full benefit entitlement?

CAN226U

(0=Not satisfied; 1=Satisfied; 9=Not known)

Appendix 5

CAN–R Summary scoring sheets

CAN–R
Complete assessment summary sheet

User name _____ Date of assessment _____/_____/_____

Staff name _____ Date of assessment _____/_____/_____

	Need		Informal help given		Formal help given		Formal help needed		Type of help		Amount of help
Rating	0,1,2,9		0,1,2,3,9		0,1,2,3,9		0,1,2,3,9		0,1,9		0,1,9
User/Staff rating	1U	1S	2U	2S	3U	3S	4U	4S	5U	5S	6U
1 Accommodation											
2 Food											
3 Looking after home											
4 Self-care											
5 Daytime activities											
6 Physical health											
7 Psychotic symptoms											
8 Information											
9 Psychological distress											
10 Safety to self											
11 Safety to others											
12 Alcohol											
13 Drugs											
14 Company											
15 Intimate relationships											
16 Sexual expression											
17 Child care											
18 Education											
19 Telephone											
20 Transport											
21 Money											
22 Benefits											
Number of met needs (Number of 1s)											
Number of unmet needs (Number of 2s)											
Total number of needs (Number of 1s and 2s)											
Total level of help given & needed, & satisfaction (Add scores, rate 9 as 0)											

CAN–R
User assessment summary sheet

User name _____ Date of assessment ____/____/____

Interviewer _____

	Need	Informal help given	Formal help given	Formal help needed	Type of help	Amount of help
Rating	0,1,2,9	0,1,2,3,9	0,1,2,3,9	0,1,2,3,9	0,1,9	0,1,9
User/Staff rating	1U	2U	3U	4U	5U	6U
1 Accommodation						
2 Food						
3 Looking after home						
4 Self-care						
5 Daytime activities						
6 Physical health						
7 Psychotic symptoms						
8 Information						
9 Psychological distress						
10 Safety to self						
11 Safety to others						
12 Alcohol						
13 Drugs						
14 Company						
15 Intimate relationships						
16 Sexual expression						
17 Child care						
18 Education						
19 Telephone						
20 Transport						
21 Money						
22 Benefits						
Number of met needs (Number of 1s)						
Number of unmet needs (Number of 2s)						
Total number of needs (Number of 1s and 2s)						
Total level of help given & needed, & satisfaction (Add scores, rate 9 as 0)						

CAN-R
Staff assessment summary sheet

User name _____

Staff name _____   Date of assessment _____ / ____ / _____

	Need	Informal help given	Formal help given	Formal help needed	Type of help
Rating	0,1,2,9	0,1,2,3,9	0,1,2,3,9	0,1,2,3,9	0,1,9
User/Staff rating	1S	2S	3S	4S	5S
1 Accommodation					
2 Food					
3 Looking after home					
4 Self-care					
5 Daytime activities					
6 Physical health					
7 Psychotic symptoms					
8 Information					
9 Psychological distress					
10 Safety to self					
11 Safety to others					
12 Alcohol					
13 Drugs					
14 Company					
15 Intimate relationships					
16 Sexual expression					
17 Child care					
18 Education					
19 Telephone					
20 Transport					
21 Money					
22 Benefits					
Number of met needs (Number of 1s)					
Number of unmet needs (Number of 2s)					
Total number of needs (Number of 1s and 2s)					
Total level of help given & needed, & satisfaction (Add scores, rate 9 as 0)					

Appendix 6

Training pack

Practice vignette
5 Full vignettes, complete with notes and completed summary score sheets
3 Overheads

Practice vignette

User interview with Jeanette

Safety to self

You do have worries about killing yourself, but your mother keeps you going by being very supportive and is often in touch with you. You also know that you could contact your psychiatrist if things got really bad. However, you would like staff to check up on you, rather than you having to contact them. You therefore don't feel happy with the help you are getting at present. (Expected rating 1 3 1 2 0 0)

Safety to others

You occasionally feel very angry, but know that you would never be violent towards other people. (Expected rating 0)

Staff interview with Dr Jones

Safety to self

Jeanette has discussed her suicidal ideation with you, so you know that it is a problem. You ask her about it at each three-monthly out-patient appointment, but you would like to assess her more regularly – ideally weekly. She gets some support from her relatives, although you have the impression that they cannot cope with her worries more than about once a week. All in all, she gets the right type of help at present. (Expected rating 1 2 1 2 1)

Safety to others

Jeanette has no history of violence, but she has a lot of bottled up emotions. You think she is at risk of violence, so always check on that aspect during out-patient appointment, which is the right level of help at present. She gets no help from relatives with this. She gets the right type of help at present. (Expected rating 1 0 1 1 1)

Full vignette 1

A worked example of a summary sheet is now given, based on (fictitious) interviews with Chris, a mental health service user, and Richard, Chris's keyworker

Interview with Chris

Chris enjoys living in her hostel, though she would like to have her own accommodation, and says her keyworker, Richard, refuses to refer her. She occasionally gets "moaned at" by hostel staff to clean her bedroom, but would like some practical help from them. She does not need any help in keeping herself clean. Every day she attends a day centre, where she has a meal. All other meals are supplied at the hostel and she needs this level of help. Chris reports that the centre is boring, and makes her feelings of loneliness even worse. She does not know what she would prefer to do during the day, but is unhappy with the current arrangements. The staff have been very helpful already in arranging for her to attend (the day centre) but she feels that she would need a lot of help with finding more enjoyable things to do. She is often lonely or feels low, and rings her mother every month or so about this. Apart from that she gets no help with her difficulties from friends or relatives. She would like to talk to Richard about how she feels when she is lonely or down, but does not get the chance at present. She is physically well, and although there is nothing wrong with her thoughts or nerves, they make her have an injection. She has never felt like hitting anyone else or harming herself, and does not drink or take drugs. Chris reports that she is single and has no sex life, both of which are "okay". She has no children. Her reading is not very good, and she would like Richard to fill in forms for her, although he does not help in this way at present. Chris has to ask before she can use the pay phone in the hostel. Although the hostel staff always let her use the telephone, she would prefer her own telephone in her room. She has a bus pass, which is "wonderful". She has no difficulty budgeting, and Richard is sorting out a new benefit for her.

Interview with Richard, Chris's keyworker

Chris lives in a hostel for people with mental health problems, which is the right sort of accommodation for her. All meals are provided for her by the hostel and day centre, which is needed. Hostel staff occasionally help tidy her bedroom (which Chris needs), but she keeps herself clean. She attends a day centre most days, and would be lonely if not attending. Chris has been quite happy in the last month. Physically she is well. She has been diagnosed as having a psychotic illness, which is reviewed by her psychiatrist every three months. Richard would like to give Chris a comprehensive education about her illness, but whenever he tries to talk to Chris about this she says she does not want to hear anything about it. However, sometimes Chris says that her mother told her she is not ill, so Richard is not sure if Chris discusses her mental health with her mother. Apart from this, Richard believes that she has no friends or contact with family. She is not suicidal or violent, and does not drink or take drugs. Richard believes (but is not sure) that Chris does not want a relationship with anyone at the moment, and he has never asked if Chris has any sexual problems. Chris has no children. Because Chris cannot read, either Richard or the hostel staff fill in any forms for her. Richard is not sure whether this is the most appropriate help with literacy, but is unsure what else could be done. She has a bus pass and access to a telephone at the hostel when she asks, which meets her needs in these areas. She finds it hard to save money, but "gets by". Richard has recently applied on her behalf for Disability Living Allowance.

Notes

Domain 5 (Daytime activities)

User's assessment of need = 2
Despite attending a day centre she says that she feels bored and is unhappy with current arrangements.

User's assessment of formal help needed = 3
Although she does not know what type of help she needs, she does appear to accept that she needs a high level of help.

Domain 7 (Psychotic symptoms)

User's assessment of need = 0
Although she says that she has an injection, she does not believe that there is anything wrong with her thoughts or nerves.

Staff assessment of formal help needed = 1
Although this is not specifically stated, it is implied that she is receiving as much help as needed.

CAN–R
Complete assessment summary sheet

User name	Chris	Date of assessment	11 / 11 / 1998
Staff name	Richard, keyworker	Date of assessment	11 / 11 / 1998

	Need		Informal help given		Formal help given		Formal help needed		Type of help		Amount of help
Rating	0,1,2,9		0,1,2,3,9		0,1,2,3,9		0,1,2,3,9		0,1,9		0,1,9
User/Staff rating	1U	1S	2U	2S	3U	3S	4U	4S	5U	5S	6U
1 Accommodation	1	1	0	0	3	3	2	3	0	1	1
2 Food	1	1	0	0	3	3	3	3	1	1	1
3 Looking after home	1	1	0	0	1	2	2	2	0	1	0
4 Self-care	0	0									
5 Daytime activities	2	1	0	0	0	3	3	3	0	1	1
6 Physical health	0	0									
7 Psychotic symptoms	0	1		9		1		1		1	
8 Information	0	2		9		0		3		1	
9 Psychological distress	1	0	1		0		1		0		0
10 Safety to self	0	0									
11 Safety to others	0	0									
12 Alcohol	0	0									
13 Drugs	0	0									
14 Company	2	1	1	9	0	3	1	3	0	1	0
15 Intimate relationships	0	0									
16 Sexual expression	0	9									
17 Child care	0	0									
18 Education	2	1	0	0	0	1	1	9	0	9	0
19 Telephone	1	1	0	0	1	1	3	1	0	1	0
20 Transport	1	1	0	0	1	1	1	1	1	1	1
21 Money	0	0									
22 Benefits	1	1	0	0	2	2	2	2	1	1	1
Number of met needs (Number of 1s)	7	10									
Number of unmet needs (Number of 2s)	3	1									
Total number of needs (Number of 1s and 2s)	10	11									
Total level of help given & needed, & satisfaction (Add scores, rate 9 as 0)			2	0	11	20	19	22	3	10	5

Full vignette 2

A worked example of a summary sheet is now given, based on (fictitious) interviews with John, a 46-year-old mental health service user, and Dr Johnson, John's psychiatrist

Interview with John

John has always lived with his mother, which he finds alright, although she wants him to move out. She makes all his meals, though John would like to have more of a range of food, because he doesn't like potatoes very much. He is not too worried about it, though, and his mother is certainly the right person to cook for him. The only help he gets from local services is a GP who won't listen to him and a psychiatrist who sees him, "to talk about my schizophrenia". His mother does the housework, but he would be quite able to do it if she didn't. She always complains that John should wash more, which he accepts is a bit of a problem, but he finds it humiliating when she runs his bath, and so would rather she moaned at him less. He doesn't know what would be better, but wants more help. During the day John normally stays in watching and cataloguing his video collection, which keeps him very busy. Physically John says he is very unwell, but is unable to say what is the matter with him – "that's the doctor's job, isn't it?". The GP does not take John's physical problems seriously, and John would like to have hospital appointments. John states assertively "I'm a schizophrenic". He sees a psychiatrist (who is very good) once every three months, which is the right length of time between appointments. He can't talk to his mother – she just gets upset. John knows all there is to know about schizophrenia. He is very happy. He would never harm himself, though he does get angry with the neighbours who play loud music late into the night. He worries that he might be violent towards them one day, and sometimes he gets so angry that he shouts at his mother, who shouts back and makes him feel worse, though occasionally she is sympathetic. The only help he wants is for someone to stop the neighbours playing their music, because he is not the one with the problem. He takes neither drugs nor alcohol, and does not want friends, because he has always been a loner and is happy with his mother. He is not in a relationship with anyone at present, because "women are always trouble". He wants nothing to do with sex, and he has no children. He reads a lot, and has no problems buying things. Although John never calls anyone, he would know how to use the telephone in an emergency. He gets a bus pass which, although he never needs to use it (because he lives near the hospital for his appointments), would be useful if he did. John is good at saving, although the benefits do not go far. He knows, however, that he gets everything that he is eligible for.

Interview with Dr Johnson

John's accommodation is fine until his mother is unable to care for him, when he will need supported accommodation. His mother makes all the food, because John cannot cook, and it is probably too late for him to learn. The same applies to the housework, and for both cooking and looking after the home

John would need considerable help from support services if his mother was not there. Hygiene is a problem, and Dr Johnson regularly prompts John to take better care of himself, as does his mother a lot of the time. However, he really needs a more structured skill-training programme, because prompting is not working. During the day John rarely leaves the house, and is engrossed with his hobby. Although not the best use of his time, this is not a problem. John occasionally imagines all sorts of physical illnesses that he has not got, and is physically well. His schizophrenia is well maintained by a three-monthly review, the correct frequency of out-patient appointments. Dr Johnson has told John a lot about his illness, but would like to have more time to talk to him about some aspects. He is not a suicide risk, and although he gets moderately anxious, he is not at risk of being violent. John does not drink or take drugs. He is socially isolated, only seeing his mother every day, and Dr Johnson has suggested several times that he attend a day centre, but John does not want to consider it. He has no interest in relationships or sex, and has no children. John is relatively literate and numerate, but Dr Johnson does not know if he can use the telephone or public transport (although he has a bus pass). John only spends money on blank videos, and so manages to save a little. He gets his full benefit entitlement.

Notes

Domain 2 (Food)	User's assessment of need = 0 Although he is not completely happy, he does not feel that it is a serious problem.
Domain 4 (Self-care)	Staff assessment of informal help = 1 Although from information provided a 2 is possible.
Domain 9 (Psychological distress)	Staff assessment of need = 0 Although described as 'moderately anxious' and 'occasionally' imagining physical illnesses, the doctor does not seem to think that there are serious problems.
Domain 20 (Transport)	Staff assessment of need = 9 Although the doctor knows that John has a bus pass, he does not know if he uses it.

CAN–R
Complete assessment summary sheet

User name _____ John _____   Date of assessment __11_ / _11_ / _1998_

Staff name _____ Dr Johnson, psychiatrist _____   Date of assessment __11_ / _11_ / _1998_

	Need		Informal help given		Formal help given		Formal help needed		Type of help		Amount of help
Rating	0,1,2,9		0,1,2,3,9		0,1,2,3,9		0,1,2,3,9		0,1,9		0,1,9
User/Staff rating	1U	1S	2U	2S	3U	3S	4U	4S	5U	5S	6U
1 Accommodation	0	0									
2 Food	0	1		3		0		0		1	
3 Looking after home	0	1		3		0		0		1	
4 Self-care	1	2	2	1	0	1	1	3	0	0	0
5 Daytime activities	0	0									
6 Physical health	2	0	0		0		2		0		0
7 Psychotic symptoms	1	1	0	0	1	1	1	1	9	1	1
8 Information	0	1		0		1		2		1	
9 Psychological distress	0	0									
10 Safety to self	0	0									
11 Safety to others	2	0	1			0		9		9	9
12 Alcohol	0	0									
13 Drugs	0	0									
14 Company	0	2		3		1		2		0	
15 Intimate relationships	0	0									
16 Sexual expression	0	0									
17 Child care	0	0									
18 Education	0	0									
19 Telephone	0	9									
20 Transport	1	9	0		1		1		1		1
21 Money	0	0									
22 Benefits	0	0									
Number of met needs (Number of 1s)	3	4									
Number of unmet needs (Number of 2s)	2	2									
Total number of needs (Number of 1s and 2s)	5	6									
Total level of help given & needed, & satisfaction (Add scores, rate 9 as 0)			3	10	2	4	5	8	1	4	2

Full vignette 3

A worked example of a summary sheet is now given, based on (fictitious) interviews with Anna, a mental health service user, and Dr Hughes, Anna's psychiatrist

Interview with Anna

Anna was admitted to an acute psychiatric ward three weeks ago. When not in hospital she lives in a council flat with her partner Edward. When at home she does her own cooking, shopping and housework, but does not currently feel that she can manage them. Edward does nothing to help and goes out drinking most days. She has no problems looking after herself. On the ward she has an occupational therapy programme, but is not interested in any of it apart from cooking and so does not attend. When at home she is busy looking after the house and three children. She suffers from diabetes and has a lot of problems with it, having been admitted to hospital unconscious several times, usually if she has been drinking at a party. She knows she ought to go to a diabetic clinic near where she lives but often forgets, or is too busy. Edward knows about giving her glucose if she is feeling unwell but he is not around all the time so does not remind her about her insulin. Anna has been hearing God's voice telling her that she is wicked and should take all her lithium tablets. She is usually on an injection and lithium. She sees a psychiatrist every month but thinks that this is too often and does not always turn up. She is supposed to get her injection from the hospital but for the past few weeks she has been missing this. Edward had been trying to persuade her to go but this makes her angry. She also feels angry because she feels that all her psychiatrist does is to give her drugs. She does not know what these are for and would like more information and some psychotherapy. She often gets very depressed, usually when she is alone with the baby, who has problems with feeding. At these times she feels desperate and just before her admission took all her lithium tablets. Her health visitor is helpful practically and comes to see her a few times a week, to advise about the baby. The only other person who calls is her social worker but she often does not let her in as she is worried that the social worker will say she is not able to look after her children properly. She would never be aggressive to anyone. She only drinks occasionally and never uses any drugs. Anna never feels lonely; in fact she would sometimes like more time to herself as she feels she never gets a break from the children. She has a friend with children who will occasionally babysit. She does have problems in her relationship with Edward, mostly because of his drinking, and she would like some help with this, but is not sure what. She did not wish to discuss their sex life. Usually Anna can look after the children, but there is no one to care for them when she is in hospital. She is in contact with her mother, who is sympathetic and advises Anna to see her doctor when she is unwell. But she lives too far away to offer any practical help. Anna can read and write. She has a telephone but when she gets very low she does not use it because when she picks it up she hears the unpleasant voice telling her that she is evil. She is currently not using the phone because of this. Anna travels on the bus and would like a bus pass. She is always short of money, as she gives it to Edward. She knows that this is a mistake but does not want any help with her money, and knows that she is getting all of her benefits.

Interview with Dr Hughes

Anna's accommodation is satisfactory, and when well she has no problems with managing her home and cooking, but Dr Hughes does not know what he could do at the moment. She has a major problem with obesity but will not follow any of the suggested diets. Edward is of little help with anything and is quite a troublesome influence as he drinks excessively and encourages Anna to drink, which exacerbates her problems with diabetic control. She takes her insulin erratically, especially when unwell. She really needs a diabetic nurse to visit regularly but this is not available. Anna has enough to do during the day looking after her children. It would be helpful if there was a nursery placement for the youngest child, to take some of the strain off Anna, but staff have not been able to find a nursery place. There is a lot of concern about her ability to look after the children and as she has frequent relapses they have been in and out of care. Edward is not the father, and in any case social services are not happy about the children being left with him. Anna frequently has psychotic relapses, mostly because of non-compliance. She does have a community psychiatric nurse who visits monthly but this should probably be more frequent, and the community psychiatric nurse needs to start giving the depot rather than it being given at a depot clinic. Dr Hughes has explained at length to Anna about her illness and the need for medication, but he is not sure that she has taken it in, and she does not always accept she is ill. Anna is quite a risk to herself when psychotic as she often acts on the voices' suggestion about overdosing, but she has never threatened to harm anyone else. She needs to be in hospital at present for this reason. Anna has no problems with company. Her relationship with Edward is not helpful because he drinks, but she does not want to leave him and Dr Hughes is pessimistic about seeing them as a couple because he feels that Edward would not comply, though this has not been offered. Anna does not drink excessively, but when she does have a drink it causes her problems because it interferes with her diabetic control. Anna can read and write and has no problems travelling. Dr Hughes feels that she will need some specific help with her anxiety about using the telephone at home with a behavioural approach from either her community psychiatric nurse or a psychologist. This problem can be quite handicapping. Budgeting is a major problem because she gives money to Edward and Dr Hughes feels that it is going to be necessary to tackle this by getting a social worker involved in trying to supervise her payment of essential bills. She has had a recent evaluation of her benefits by her social worker.

Notes

Domain 2, 3, 4	Staff assessment of need = 9
(Food, Looking after home, Self-care)	Although she normally can manage these areas it is important to rate whether there has been a problem during the last month.

CAN–R
Complete assessment summary sheet

User name	Anna	Date of assessment	11 / 11 / 1998
Staff name	Dr Hughes, psychiatrist	Date of assessment	11 / 11 / 1998

	Need		Informal help given		Formal help given		Formal help needed		Type of help		Amount of help
Rating	0,1,2,9		0,1,2,3,9		0,1,2,3,9		0,1,2,3,9		0,1,9		0,1,9
User/Staff rating	1U	1S	2U	2S	3U	3S	4U	4S	5U	5S	6U
1 Accommodation	0	0									
2 Food	1	9	0		3		3		9		9
3 Looking after home	1	9	0		3		3		9		9
4 Self-care	0	9									
5 Daytime activities	0	0									
6 Physical health	2	2	0	0	1	1	2	2	0	0	0
7 Psychotic symptoms	1	1	2	0	3	3	1	3	0	1	0
8 Information	2	1	0	0	0	2	2	3	0	1	0
9 Psychological distress	1	9	9		2		2		9		9
10 Safety to self	1	1	0	0	3	3	9	3	9	1	9
11 Safety to others	0	0									
12 Alcohol	0	2		0		0		1		0	
13 Drugs	0	9									
14 Company	0	0									
15 Intimate relationships	2	2	0	0	0	0	9	9	0	0	0
16 Sexual expression	0	9									
17 Child care	1	2	0	9	1	2	1	9	9	0	9
18 Education	0	0									
19 Telephone	2	2	0	0	0	0	9	2	9	0	9
20 Transport	2	0	0		0		1		0		0
21 Money	2	2	0	0	0	0	0	2	1	0	1
22 Benefits	0	1		0		3		9		9	
Number of met needs (Number of 1s)	6	4									
Number of unmet needs (Number of 2s)	6	6									
Total number of needs (Number of 1s and 2s)	12	10									
Total level of help given & needed, & satisfaction (Add scores, rate 9 as 0)			2	0	16	14	15	16	1	3	1

Full vignette 4

A worked example of a summary sheet is now given, based on (fictitious) interviews with Peter, a 63-year-old mental health service user, and Jackie, Peter's keyworker

Interview with Peter

Peter has been happy living with his sister, Mary, in her flat for the past 25 years. Mary does all the housework and cooking, although Peter gets lunch at the day centre on Fridays. The day centre isn't local to Peter but he can get there using his bus pass, and meeting up with old friends makes the travel worthwhile. On the other days of the week he occupies himself by gardening and going to the pub most evenings, where he drinks three or four pints with the other regulars. Peter keeps himself clean but describes himself as never having been "fashion conscious" and is appreciative of the fact that his sister takes care of all the laundry and puts out clean clothes for him each day. In turn he helps with the maintenance of the flat and two weeks ago he put up some shelves in the kitchen. Unfortunately this hurt his back and Mary had to call out the GP. The doctor prescribed rest and offered him another appointment but Peter didn't attend it as he felt fine within a couple of days. He also sees a doctor at the psychiatric hospital every three months and his sister reminds him about the appointment dates. He likes seeing the psychiatrist, having known her for some years, and she usually asks him how he has been getting on and prescribes tablets which have reduced the voices that he hears. She also has a tendency to nag him about his drinking. Peter knows about his medication and that he shouldn't drink with it, but he is not prepared to sacrifice his social life and he knows lots of people who drink more than he does. He reports that drink doesn't make him aggressive, that he is actually a placid and quite contented person and furthermore that he has never needed to take drugs to achieve that state, unlike a lot of the "youngsters in this day and age". Peter has never married or had children and feels that he is too old to bother with a girlfriend and hasn't got the energy "for that sort of thing". He is quite happy to hand over his benefit money to Mary each week for her to pay the bills and give him money as he needs it. Recently his sister told him to ask the staff at the day centre whether he could get any more money. Although Peter doesn't have problems reading, both he and Mary found it difficult to make sense of the pamphlet he was given by his keyworker Jackie. He is unhappy about the situation and says that he will ring his keyworker once he gets home.

Interview with Jackie

Peter lives with his sister in a flat which Jackie visited one month ago. It was clean but Jackie doesn't know whether Peter helps out around the house. He appears to be able to look after himself as he is always well turned out and well nourished, the latter probably due to his fortune in having a good cook for a sister. Also, Peter has lunch at the day centre once a week with a group of fellow attenders he is friends with. He travels in by bus and is happy to use his free pass to get around on his own. Jackie would like to see Peter engage more in the activities of the day centre and thinks that he would benefit from attending the men's and art groups they run. However he has declined her offer. Peter sees a psychiatrist quarterly to monitor his psychotic illness, which has been stable on neuroleptics for the last few years. Peter seems to take his medication willingly and his sister is encouraging of this. However, although he is accepting of the fact that he has a mental disorder and understands the importance of medication compliance, Jackie is rather concerned about his drinking habits. Peter would not seek to deliberately harm himself and doesn't pose a danger to others, but she has spoken to him several times about the risks of excessive drinking, particularly when combined with his medication. She believes a major problem is that the pub forms the centre of his social life. This helps to keep him from getting lonely and Jackie believes that Peter needs to receive more intensive input to restructure his social contacts around other activities. Peter has told her that Mary goes on at him about his drinking and Jackie is frustrated that she doesn't have the time to do more. Peter doesn't take drugs, has no children and has no problems with numeracy or literacy. Indeed recently he was enquiring about his benefit entitlement and was able to calculate his present weekly income. He said that his sister had been asking questions about whether he would be entitled to anything more. Jackie gave them a booklet to read in their own time which would explain the different types of allowances. Jackie does not know if Peter has any specific sexual difficulties, but believes that he wants a partner and thinks that the weekly men's group would be an ideal opportunity for him to discuss his feelings about this. She doubts whether he can talk to his sister about relationships or sex. However, in general he has been in good health and spirits over the last month.

Notes

Domain 2,3 (Food, Looking after home)	User's assessment of need = 1 Although from the information supplied it is not possible to be certain, it appears as if he would have a problem with food and household tasks if his sister was not there.
Domain 6 (Physical health)	User's assessment of need = 0 Although he did have backache, this was short lived and not a serious problem.
Domain 12 (Alcohol)	User's assessment of need = 0 Although he does drink heavily, he does not see it as a problem himself.
Domain 22 (Benefit)	Staff assessment of formal help needed = 1 Jackie appears to think that the booklet is adequate help.

CAN–R
Complete assessment summary sheet

User name _____Peter_____ Date of assessment __11__ / __11__ / __1998__

Staff name _____Jackie, keyworker_____ Date of assessment __11__ / __11__ / __1998__

	Need		Informal help given		Formal help given		Formal help needed		Type of help		Amount of help
Rating	0,1,2,9		0,1,2,3,9		0,1,2,3,9		0,1,2,3,9		0,1,9		0,1,9
User/Staff rating	1U	1S	2U	2S	3U	3S	4U	4S	5U	5S	6U
1 Accommodation	0	0									
2 Food	1	9	3		1		1		1		1
3 Looking after home	1	9	3		0		0		1		1
4 Self-care	0	9									
5 Daytime activities	0	1		0		1		2		0	
6 Physical health	0	9									
7 Psychotic symptoms	1	1	1	1	1	1	1	1	1	1	1
8 Information	9	0									
9 Psychological distress	0	0									
10 Safety to self	0	0									
11 Safety to others	0	0									
12 Alcohol	0	2		1		1		2		0	
13 Drugs	0	0									
14 Company	0	1		3		0		2		0	
15 Intimate relationships	0	2		0		0		2		0	
16 Sexual expression	0	9									
17 Child care	0	0									
18 Education	0	0									
19 Telephone	9	9									
20 Transport	1	9	0		1		1		1		1
21 Money	1	0	2		0		0		1		1
22 Benefits	2	1	1	0	1	1	2	1	0	1	0
Number of met needs (Number of 1s)	5	4									
Number of unmet needs (Number of 2s)	1	2									
Total number of needs (Number of 1s and 2s)	6	6									
Total level of help given & needed, & satisfaction (Add scores, rate 9 as 0)			10	5	4	4	5	10	5	2	5

Full vignette 5

A worked example of a summary sheet is now given, based on (fictitious) interviews with George, a mental health service user, and George's GP

Interview with George

George rents a flat and cooks for himself, although mainly he makes snacks for himself, or buys take-away food. He cleans his flat when he feels it needs to be done. More importantly, he does not feel very safe in his flat because the front door doesn't lock properly. However, he doesn't want to move as he knows the area and has a neighbour who has always been good to him. He is able to look after his personal hygiene and does his own laundry. He is supposed to go to a sheltered employment scheme four mornings a week but attends irregularly because he finds it boring. He wants to work but doesn't think that he can get a job in the current economic climate. He would like to know who can help him with this problem. George feels his physical health is good, although he knows he is overweight. He smokes 40 cigarettes a day and his GP keeps telling him to cut down. He has to see his GP every two months for medication for his "nerves", which he knows he needs, although at times he forgets to take it. The medication also helps to stop the voices he hears. One of his neighbours who he knows asks him if he is taking his medication from time to time. In the last month he has felt OK, although he does get depressed at times. Two years ago he tried to jump under a train, " a voice made me do it". He does worry that he might harm someone, not because he wants to, but "because of the voices" – two months ago a voice did try to make him do this, so the neighbour called the GP. He was taken to hospital and came out two weeks ago. He feels much better now. He does not drink alcohol or take any drugs except those from the doctor. He does get lonely but he does not want any close friends, in the past people who he thought were his friends have stolen money from him and he doesn't trust anyone anymore. However, he does go to a drop-in cafe nearby a couple of times a week for a cup of tea and some food. He finds the weekends particularly difficult and thinks that the drop-in should be open for a few hours on a Saturday and Sunday. At times he would like a girlfriend, although he thinks that it would be too much trouble and thinks the drugs have "slowed me up". He doesn't talk to anyone about this, although he thinks that perhaps he would like to but he's not sure who. He has no children. George enjoys reading and is thinking of doing an English course at evening classes next year. He is not behind with his rent but currently he is paying for food and cigarettes on credit with the shopkeeper across the road. He isn't sure whether he is getting all the benefits that he is entitled to and he would like someone to check this. He has a bus pass and travels locally and occasionally into the centre of the city. There is no telephone in his flat but he never needs the phone; the staff at the employment scheme let him use their telephone on the occasions when he does need it.

George's GP

George lives in a flat which is very insecure with only a flimsy lock on the front door. The estate isn't safe and the GP is concerned for his safety because George does tend to let people into his flat too easily. On a visit to his flat two months ago when George was admitted to hospital, the flat was very dirty and smelt. The flat needed redecorating and cleaning and a social worker has now been appointed to George's case since his hospital admission. It is the GP's opinion that George should live in supported accommodation because he is very vulnerable. His personal hygiene is adequate. With regard to daytime activities the GP knows that George goes to a sheltered employment scheme a couple of mornings a week, which isn't stimulating enough for George but is the best option available. George has not worked in open employment for over 10 years and the GP doubts whether he could hold down a job. Physically, George's health is OK although he is overweight and his blood pressure needs to be checked regularly. The GP sees George every six weeks and prescribes him oral medication, which is acceptable to George, although there are lapses in taking it which usually precipitates a hospital admission. There have been four admissions in the last 12 months, the most recent one being two months ago. The GP would like more follow-up from the hospital and thinks that George needs a community psychiatric nurse to provide more support. He thinks that George does get depressed at times because he will usually come to the surgery for no particular reason and want to just chat to the GP. There are no alcohol or drug misuse problems. George has very little contact with his family and as far as the GP is aware he has no close friends, although there are people who come and go at his flat, which concerns the GP. He has never heard George talk of any long-standing relationships. It is because George is so isolated that the GP thinks that he needs to live in a more supported environment. George does have one interest: he reads and picks up books from second-hand stalls. He needs assistance with budgeting as he is currently paying for his food and cigarettes on credit from the shop across the road, although the GP is not sure whether George would accept this help. He thinks that George has a bus pass but isn't sure and does not know whether he is receiving the benefits he is entitled to. Hopefully the social worker will be investigating this. George doesn't have a telephone and the GP doesn't know whether he can use one because he has never asked George about this.

Notes

| Domain 7 | Staff assessment of formal help needed = 3 |
| (Psychotic symptoms) | GP clearly believes that he needs more help than he is currently receiving. |

| Domain 14 | Staff assessment of formal help given = 9 |
| (Company) | GP appears unaware that George attends drop-in. |

| Domain 19 | User's assessment of need = 0 |
| (Telephone) | Although he does not have access to a telephone he specifically says that he does not need a telephone. |

| Domain 22 | Staff assessment of formal help given = 0 |
| (Benefits) | The social worker has not yet investigated the benefits entitlement, although this might be planned. |

CAN–R
Complete assessment summary sheet

User name	George	Date of assessment	11 / 11 / 1998
Staff name	George's GP	Date of assessment	11 / 11 / 1998

	Need		Informal help given		Formal help given		Formal help needed		Type of help		Amount of help
Rating	0,1,2,9		0,1,2,3,9		0,1,2,3,9		0,1,2,3,9		0,1,9		0,1,9
User/Staff rating	1U	1S	2U	2S	3U	3S	4U	4S	5U	5S	6U
1 Accommodation	2	2	0	0	0	9	2	3	0	0	0
2 Food	0	9									
3 Looking after home	0	2		0		0		2		0	
4 Self-care	0	0									
5 Daytime activities	2	1	0	0	2	2	1	2	1	0	0
6 Physical health	0	1		0		2		2		1	
7 Psychotic symptoms	1	2	1	0	2	2	2	3	1	0	9
8 Information	9	9									
9 Psychological distress	0	1		0		1		2		0	
10 Safety to self	0	0									
11 Safety to others	1	0	1		2		2		1		9
12 Alcohol	0	0									
13 Drugs	0	0									
14 Company	1	2	9	0	2	9	3	3	1	0	1
15 Intimate relationships	0	9									
16 Sexual expression	9	9									
17 Child care	0	9									
18 Education	0	0									
19 Telephone	0	9									
20 Transport	1	9	0		1		1		1		1
21 Money	1	2	9	0	0	0	9	1	9	0	9
22 Benefits	2	2	9	0	9	0	3	2	9	0	9
Number of met needs (Number of 1s)	5	3									
Number of unmet needs (Number of 2s)	3	6									
Total number of needs (Number of 1s and 2s)	8	9									
Total level of help given & needed, & satisfaction (Add scores, rate 9 as 0)			2	0	9	7	14	20	5	1	2

Issues to consider

- What is need?

    "The requirements of individuals to enable them to achieve, maintain or restore an acceptable level of social independence or quality of life."

    National Health Service and
    Community Care Act (1990)

- Overmet, met and unmet need

- Perceptions of need

Section 1

- Trigger questions

- Does it measure need, existence of intervention or effectiveness of intervention?

- What is an intervention?

- How to rate when there is an intervention but no perceived need

- How to rate when there is a:
  - totally effective intervention
  - partly effective intervention
  - totally ineffective intervention

Sections 2 & 3

- Level of help and anchor points

- What about when the intervention is perceived as not helping?

- Difference between help given and needed

Section 4

- What is the difference?

Appendix 7

CAN reliability and validity

Reprinted from the *British Journal of Psychiatry*

BRITISH JOURNAL OF PSYCHIATRY (1995), 167, 589–595

The Camberwell Assessment of Need:

the validity and reliability of an instrument to assess

the needs of people with severe mental illness

MICHAEL PHELAN, MIKE SLADE, GRAHAM THORNICROFT,
GRAHAM DUNN, FRANK HOLLOWAY, TIL WYKES, GERALDINE STRATHDEE,
LINDA LOFTUS, PAUL McCRONE and PETER HAYWARD

Background   People with severe mental illness often have a complex mixture of clinical and social needs. The Camberwell Assessment of Need (CAN) is a new instrument which has been designed to provide a comprehensive assessment of these needs. There are two versions of the instrument: the clinical version has been designed to be used by staff to plan patients' care; whereas the research version is primarily a mental health service evaluation tool. The CAN has been designed to assist local authorities to fulfil their statutory obligations under the National Health Service and Community Care Act 1990 to assess needs for community services.

Method   A draft version of the instrument was designed by the authors. Modifications were made following comments from mental health experts and a patient survey. Patients ($n=49$) and staff ($n=60$) were then interviewed, using the amended version, to assess the inter-rater and test–retest reliability of the instrument.

Results   The mean number of needs identified per patient ranged from 7.55 to 8.64. Correlations of the inter-rater and test–retest reliability of the total number of needs identified by staff were 0.99 and 0.78 respectively. The percentage of complete agreement on individual items ranged from 100–81.6% (inter-rater) and 100–58.1% (test–retest).

Conclusions   The study suggests that the CAN is a valid and reliable instrument for assessing the needs of people with severe mental illness. It is easily learnt by staff from a range of professional backgrounds, and a complete assessment took, on average, around 25 minutes.

In Britain, the importance of assessing need for services has been recognised in recent government legislation (House of Commons, 1990), but in the field of mental health there is widespread uncertainty about how this should best be done, and confusion and conflict among different professional groups is common (Holloway, 1994). Official guidelines state that need is a complex concept, defined as:

> "the requirements of individuals to enable them to achieve, maintain or restore an acceptable level of social independence or quality of life, as defined by the particular care agency or authority". (Department of Health Social Services Inspectorate, 1991, p. 10)

Other definitions of need have been proposed. Maslow (1954) set out a hierarchy of universal needs as a model for understanding human actions. Bradshaw (1972) examined need from a sociological perspective, and distinguished between normative, felt, expressed and comparative need. Changes in the concept since the 1960s, in terms of health service planning, have been described by Stevens & Gabbay (1991), who concluded that a suitable working definition was "the ability to benefit in some way from health care". For people with a severe mental illness it is appropriate to expand this definition to include social care as well as health care.

Numerous instruments have been developed to assess the level of social functioning and attainment of social roles among people with severe mental illness (Phelan *et al*, 1994). Such instruments have been designed to measure and record levels of disability without regard to whether the disabilities can be reduced. Although the results of such assessments may indicate where help is needed, this is not their prime function.

Conversely, the Medical Research Council's Needs for Care Assessment (NCA) was designed to identify areas of remediable need. Need, in the NCA, exists where a patient's level of functioning has fallen below, or threatens to fall below, some minimum specified level, and for which there is effective care (Brewin *et al*, 1987). Results from a number of studies suggest that the instrument has good reliability if used by suitably trained investigators (Brewin & Wing, 1993). Difficulties have arisen when the instrument was used for measuring need among long-term in-patients (Pryce *et al*, 1993) and homeless mentally ill people (Hogg & Marshall, 1992).

This paper describes the development of a new needs assessment schedule which fulfils the statutory obligations of services to conduct comprehensive needs assessments, and which can assist the routine care and treatment of people with severe mental illness by encouraging systematic and regular needs assessments to shape care plans. In addition it is hoped that it proves to be a powerful tool in evaluative research.

DEVELOPMENT OF THE CAMBERWELL ASSESSMENT OF NEED

Four principles shaped the development of the Camberwell Assessment of Need (CAN). Firstly, is the premise that everyone has needs, and that although people with mental illness have some specific needs, most of their needs are similar to those of people not suffering from mental illness. The CAN reflects this notion by incorporating a wide range of human needs, such as shelter and the company of other people, as well as those specific to people suffering from mental illness. Secondly, people with mental illness may have multiple needs, which are not recognised by mental health services. Therefore, a priority for the CAN is to identify, rather than describe in depth, serious needs, since more detailed and specialist assessments can be conducted in specific areas when required. Thirdly, needs assessment should be both an integral part of routine clinical practice and a component of service evaluation, so the instrument should be easily learned and practical to use for a wide range of clinical staff. Finally, we do not accept that needs should be defined by staff alone. We have based the CAN on a model of need as a subjective concept, accepting that frequently there will be differing, but equally valid perceptions about the presence or absence of a specific need (Slade, 1994). We expected that staff and patient views about need would differ, and believed that their views should be recorded separately, rather than amalgamated into a joint rating. In clinical or in research practice, therefore, the ratings of need can be completed by staff, by the patient, or by both.

We designed the CAN to be quick and easy to use, and to apply to anyone with a severe mental illness. The specific criteria we set before designing the instrument were that it should:

(a) have adequate psychometric properties

(b) be completed within 30 minutes

(c) be usable by a wide range of professionals

(d) be suitable for both routine clinical practice and research

(e) be easily learned and used, without formal training

(f) incorporate both patients' and staff views of needs

(g) measure both met and unmet need

(h) measure the level of help received from friends or relatives, as well as from statutory services.

One version of the instrument could not fulfil the needs of both clinical and research users, so we designed separate versions: the clinical version (CAN-C) and the research version (CAN-R). The small, but important differences between the two versions are described below. Decisions about which areas of need should be included within the CAN were modified following comments received from experts and users (see below). The final 22 items included are:

(a) accommodation

(b) food

(c) household skills

(d) self-care

(e) occupation

(f) physical health

(g) psychotic symptoms

(h) information about condition and treatment

(i) psychological distress

(j) safety to self

(k) safety to others

(l) alcohol

(m) drugs

(n) company of others

(o) intimate relationships

(p) sexual expression

(q) child care

(r) basic education

(s) telephone

(t) transport

(u) money

(v) welfare benefits.

The CAN follows an identical structure for all the areas, and each area of need includes four sections. The first section establishes whether there is a need, by asking about difficulties in that area. Responses are rated on a three-point scale: 0=no serious problem; 1=no serious problem or moderate problem because of continuing intervention (met need); 2=current serious problem (unmet need). Section 2 asks about help received from friends, relatives and other informal carers. Section 3 asks about how much help the person is getting, and how much help he/she needs from local statutory services. All ratings of level of help are on a four-point scale: 0=none; 1=low; 2=moderate; 3=high. Guidelines are given to help rate each level. The research and clinical CANs differ in the fourth section: CAN-C has sections to record the views of the user about the type of help that/he she requires and to outline a care plan with a review date and named professional for each point; CAN-R has two specific questions, asking whether the person is getting the right type of help for his/her problem, and whether he/she is satisfied with the amount of help that he/she is getting.

Analysis

For the validity and reliability studies, data were analysed using the Statistical Package for Social Sciences (Windows version 6.0; SPSS, 1993) and Confidence Interval Analysis (CIA; Gardner et al, 1991) software. CAN-R was used for the reliability study, but the results are applicable to both versions since data are presented for the first three sections of the instrument, which are common to both versions. Confidence intervals (95%) were calculated for all mean values. The extent of agreement between discrete variables was examined by calculating the percentage of complete agreement and Cohen's Kappa coefficient (Cohen, 1960). Correlations are given for continuous variables.

Validity

Face validity

The CAN appears to have face validity. The Flesch reading score is 65, which is the "preferred level for most readers", and the average word length is 1.58 syllables, indicating that "most readers could comprehend the vocabulary" (Grammatik Software, 1992). Clinicians and researchers in Britain and other European countries have consistently commented that it covers the range of difficulties faced by people with severe mental illness.

Consensual validity

A draft version of the instrument was sent for comments to 50 experienced professionals in the fields of social work, psychiatry, psychology, psychiatric nursing and occupational therapy. The consensus was that there was a requirement for a needs assessment instrument, and that the CAN would be useful and relevant. On the basis of specific comments from this survey, numerous minor changes and some major changes were incorporated into the final instrument. In particular, two extra items were added – the need for sexual expression and the need for an intimate relationship.

Content validity

A parallel survey was conducted of 59 people with severe mental illness who were either current in-patients or attending a psychiatric day-hospital. All topics were rated as being at least moderately important, indicating that the instrument is free from item bias. Accommodation was rated as the most important need, and help with drugs as the least important. No additional areas of need were identified by more than two respondents.

Criteria

The lack of objective external criteria makes it difficult to establish concurrent validity. The relationship between scores on the Global Assessment of Functioning Scale (GAF) of DSM–IV (American Psychiatric Association, 1994), measuring social, occupational and psychological functioning, and need was explored. Data from the reliability study were used, and details of the study sample are given below.

When individual item scores were compared with the total GAF disability rating, a mixed picture emerges, reflecting the complex interaction between service provision, disability and need. The individual need which was most closely associated with a low level of global functioning, as measured by the GAF, was the need for help with self-care. However, even for this item the correlation was weak (r=−0.39, P=0.002). For other items a need was associated with higher global functioning; this was most apparent with a need for child care (r=0.29, P=0.02). Many other individual items were not associated with levels of global functioning on their own. Some needs (e.g. help with daytime activities) were common among all the cohort reflecting the universal importance of this area for people with a severe mental illness, regardless of individual levels of functioning. Other less common needs (e.g. protection from self-harm) are specific problems for certain people, and not individually related to their overall level of functioning.

In order to obtain a rating that could be more meaningfully compared with the global functioning rating of the GAF, an aggregated score of seven needs, reflecting the domains of disability measured by the GAF (household skills, self-care, psychotic symptoms, psychological distress, risk of self-harm, danger to others and social contact) was calculated. This aggregated score was correlated with GAF ratings (r=−0.51, P<0.001).

Reliability

The reliability study was designed to allow assessment of both inter-rater and test–retest reliability. Sixty patients were enrolled for the reliability study; details of the study sample are given in Table 1. Initial staff interviews were conducted for all selected patients (n=60). Staff came from a variety of professional backgrounds (psychiatric, nursing, psychology, occupational therapy and housing) and all acted as keyworkers for the patients. Patients and their keyworkers were interviewed separately with both the interviewer and an observer rating responses. During the interview basic sociodemographic, service use and diagnostic details were collected, and the staff

member was asked to rate the user on the unidimensional 0–90 GAF scale.

Forty-nine (82%) of the patients were able to be interviewed (t1). There were no statistically significant differences between responders and non-responders with regards to age, sex, ethnicity, living situation, service contact, clinical diagnosis or GAF ratings. Forty-one patient–staff pairs were randomly selected to be re-interviewed 1 week after the initial interview (t2), and again all staff were successfully interviewed and 31 (76%) of the patients were interviewed. Mean length of contact

was 22.1 (95% CI 14.2–30.0) months, with 8.9 (95% CI 6.7–11.1) contacts per month. The patients were all in regular contact with an inner-city mental health service, and suffered from a severe mental illness.

At the first interview the mean total number of needs identified was 7.55 (95% CI 6.41–8.6) by staff (n=60) and 8.64 (95% CI 7.26–10.0) by patients (n=49). It is important to note that although staff and patients identified approximately the same number of needs, they may not have rated the same needs. The agreement between staff and patient ratings are examined

Table 1 Characteristic of patients interviewed for the CAN reliability study (n=60)

	n	%
Mean age: years	48.3	(95% CI 45.0–51.6)
Sex		
Male	37	62
Female	23	38
Ethnicity		
White	49	82
Black-Caribbean	6	10
Black-African	5	8
Marital status		
Single	38	63
Married	8	13
Divorced	12	20
Widowed	2	3
Living situation		
Alone	22	37
Partner	7	12
With other relatives	8	13
With others	23	38
Service contact (time since first contact with psychiatric services)		
0–5 years	3	5
6–10 years	8	13
11–15 years	8	13
16–20 years	9	15
>20 years	32	53
Mean number of previous admissions	5.5	(95% CI 4.3–6.7)
Status at time of interviews		
Out-patient	26	43
In-patient	14	23
Day patient	20	33
Clinical diagnosis		
Schizophrenia	33	55
Manic–depressive psychosis	8	13
Schizoaffective disorder	4	7
Personality disorder	4	7
Non-psychotic depression	3	5
Other	8	13
GAF mean	52.7	(95% CI 49.0–56.4)

in more detail in a subsequent paper, Slade *et al* (1995).

Correlations between summary scores were calculated to indicate inter-rater and test–retest reliability. There was a high level of agreement between raters at t1 (r=0.99 and 0.98 for patient and staff ratings respectively, $P<0.01$), and moderate agreement between t1 and t2, (r=0.78 and 0.71 for patient and staff ratings respectively, $P<0.001$).

Table 2 shows the level of needs assessed for each item of the CAN by staff at the first interview. In most of the areas a significant proportion of the sample had met or partially met needs, and only a minority had serious unmet needs, possibly reflecting the high levels of staff contact for most of the sample. The need which was least often identified by the staff was help with drug use, with five patients (8% of the sample) being rated as having a problem in this area. About two-thirds of the sample were receiving some help with obtaining food, and more than four-fifths were receiving help with daytime activities.

For most of the items, staff indicated whether the patient had needs, but for sexual expression and welfare benefits, up to one-quarter of staff did not know whether a need existed.

Inter-rater and test–retest reliability was examined for each individual item of the CAN. Table 3 shows the percentage of complete agreement and kappa coefficient for section 1 (assessment of need present) for both staff and patient ratings. Both these measures indicate good agreement between the two raters at the time of the first interview. The percentage of complete agreement between the first and second interviews was on the whole lower, but still indicates substantial agreement for the majority of items. Kappa coefficients for some of the test–retest items were very low (e.g. telephone, money). Examination of the raw data revealed that this was primarily due to a substantial skew in the distributions of the ratings. This difficulty with misleading kappa coefficients is discussed in detail by Feinstein & Cicchetti (1990).

Sections 2 and 3 of the instrument, measuring the help received from friends and relatives, and the help needed and received from staff, respectively, are only completed if a need is identified in section 1. Therefore, the assessment of the reliability of these sections for individual items is hampered by low numbers, and results need to be treated with caution. The mean correlations for all the items are listed in Table 4. The low test–retest figures for section 2 (level of help received from friends or relatives) and section 3.2 (level of help needed from staff) suggest some instability.

We also timed 97 CAN assessments, and the mean time for patient and staff interviews were 16.2 and 9.4 minutes respectively (mean total time 25.6 minutes).

DISCUSSION

The results of this study indicate that the CAN goes a long way in achieving the criteria of instrument adequacy, set prior

Table 2 Staff (*n*=60) assessment of level of need for 22 items of the CAN

Item	No serious need		Met or partially met need		Serious unmet need		Not known	
	n	%	*n*	%	*n*	%	*n*	%
Accommodation	33	55	26	43	0		I	2
Food	21	35	39	65	0		0	
Household skills	39	65	17	28	0		4	7
Self-care	41	68	18	30	I	2	0	
Occupation	10	17	50	83	0		0	
Physical health	37	62	23	38	0		0	
Psychotic symptoms	22	37	36	60	2	3	0	
Information about condition and treatment	47	78	10	17	0		3	5
Psychological distress	16	27	43	72	I	2	0	
Safety to self	45	70	15	25	0		0	
Safety to others	51	85	8	13	I	2	0	
Alcohol	53	88	6	10	I	2	0	
Drugs	55	92	4	7	0		I	2
Company of others	27	45	29	48	3	5	I	2
Intimate relationships	38	63	17	28	I	2	4	7
Sexual expression[1]	33	56	II	19	0		15	25
Child care	54	90	4	7	0		2	3
Basic education	48	80	10	17	I	2	I	2
Telephone	49	82	7	12	0		4	7
Transport	27	45	28	47	3	5	2	3
Money	28	47	30	50	I	2	I	2
Welfare benefits[1]	36	60	II	18	0		12	20

1. Missing data for one case.

Table 3 Inter-rater and test–retest reliability of section 1 (assessment of need present) for the 22 items of the CAN for staff and patient interviews

| Item | Inter-rater | | | | Test–retest | | | |
| | Staff (n=60) | | Patient (n=49) | | Staff (n=41) | | Patient (n=31) | |
	% complete agreement	kappa coefficient	% complete agreement	kappa coefficient	% complete agreement	kappa coefficient	% complete agreement	kappa coefficient
Accommodation	91.7	0.84	93.9	0.88	90.2	0.81	96.8	0.93
Food	98.3	0.96	95.9	0.87	95.1	0.89	96.8	0.87
Household skills	98.3	0.96	93.9	0.89	68.3	0.38	71.0	0.48
Self-care	98.3	0.96	97.9	0.95	95.1	0.89	77.4	0.48
Occupation	91.2	0.74	95.9	0.85	95.1	0.85	96.8	0.90
Physical health	98.3	0.96	97.9	0.96	90.2	0.77	67.7	0.36
Psychotic symptoms	95.0	0.89	93.8	0.88	87.8	0.75	74.2	0.53
Information about condition and treatment	93.3	0.83	87.8	0.73	70.7	0.19	67.7	0.36
Psychological distress	96.7	0.92	95.9	0.93	75.6	0.35	71.0	0.54
Safety to self	100.0	1.00	97.9	0.94	78.0	0.35	77.4	0.52
Safety to others	100.0	1.00	93.9	0.65	85.4	0.52	83.9	0.42
Alcohol	100.0	1.00	100.0	1.00	100.0	1.00	87.1	0.44
Drugs	96.7	0.89	97.9	0.82	95.1	0.73	90.3	0.36
Company of others	95.0	0.88	93.9	0.89	63.4	0.37	77.4	0.57
Intimate relationships	88.3	0.79	91.8	0.79	78.0	0.56	83.9	0.59
Sexual expression	95.0	0.88	81.6	0.75	78.0	0.65	71.0	0.43
Child care	96.7	0.82	97.9	1.00	97.6	0.85	100.0	1
Basic education	100.0	1.00	91.8	0.82	80.5	0.52	71.0	0.43
Telephone	98.3	0.95	97.9	0.91	80.5	0.13	83.9	0.21
Transport	91.7	0.86	95.9	0.93	75.6	0.56	77.4	0.58
Money	98.3	0.97	91.8	0.86	82.9	0.67	58.1	0.23
Welfare benefits	90.0	0.81	95.9	0.93	75.6	0.54	71.0	0.49

1. Cannot be calculated due to small numbers.

to its development. It is a comprehensive and relatively brief needs assessment tool which is easy for a wide range of staff to learn and use. It incorporates the view of both staff and patients and measures both met and unmet needs. The work presented in this paper suggests that it is a valid instrument, which when used under research conditions has adequate reliability.

This study needs to be supplemented by further fieldwork in order to fully explore the qualities of the instrument. Further work is needed to explore whether the low test–retest reliability scores for some of the individual items are a reflection of changing needs between assessments, or due to flaws in the instrument itself. The main limitation of the present study was that it was conducted at one site, among a group of patients who were characterised by a high proportion of met need, which may reflect low levels of expectations

Table 4 Mean correlations between rater and observer and between t1 and t2 for the 22 items of the CAN, for sections 2, 3.1 and 3.2

			Mean r
Section 2 (help from friends or relatives)	Inter-rater	Staff ratings	0.93
		Patient ratings	0.88
	Test–retest	Staff ratings	0.34
		Patient ratings	0.36
Section 3.1 (help received from staff)	Inter-rater	Staff ratings	0.76
		Patient ratings	0.82
	Test–retest	Staff ratings	0.69
		Patient ratings	0.64
Section 3.2 (help needed from staff)	Inter-rater	Staff ratings	0.64
		Patient ratings	0.70
	Test–retest	Staff ratings	0.55
		Patient ratings	0.33

among both staff and patients, as well as high levels of service contact. Further studies are needed at different locations among other specific groups of people with severe mental illness, such as the homeless, to assess if the instrument can be successfully used with patients who have a more volatile pattern of need, and to examine its validity in other patient groups.

The research and clinical versions of the instrument (CAN-R and CAN-C) are designed for different purposes. We expect that CAN-C will be used as a routine instrument for initial assessments, the formulation of care plans and for regular case reviews CAN-R is intended to be a service evaluation instrument.

Work on the CAN is continuing. The authors have developed an electronic version of the CAN (PELICAN), allowing direct data entry and easier aggregation and analysis of data. The authors are also collaborating with colleagues who are translating the CAN into 13 European languages. There is the potential for the CAN to be customised for use with other patient groups, such as children, the elderly, and those with learning difficulties, as well as the carers of people with mental disorders. Finally, the structure of the instrument lends itself to the addition of further specific items relevant to other particular patient groups.

Now that needs assessment is recognised to be a key element of mental health care, we hope that the CAN will make a useful contribution to future patient care.

MICHAEL PHELAN, MCRPsych, MIKE SLADE, MSc, GRAHAM THORNICROFT, MRCPsych, GRAHAM DUNN, PhD, FRANK HOLLOWAY, MRCPsych, TIL WYKES, CPsyschol, GERALDINE STRATHDEE, MRCPsych, LINDA LOFTUS, MSc, PAUL McCRONE, MSc, PETER HAYWARD, PhD, Department of Psychology, Institute of Psychiatry, London

Correspondence: Dr Phelan, PRiSM, Institute of Psychiatry, De Crespigny Park, London SE5 8AF

(First received 22 November 1994, final revision 18 May 1995, accepted 19 May 1995)

REFERENCES

American Psychiatric Association (1994) *Diagnostic and Statistical Manual of Mental Disorders* (4th edn) (DSM–IV). Washington, DC: APA.

Bradshaw, J. (1972) A taxonomy of social need. In *Problems and Progress in Medical Care: Essays on Current Research* (ed. G. McLachlan) (7th series). London: Oxford University Press.

Brewin, C., Wing, J., Mangen, S., et al (1987) Principles and practice of measuring needs in the long-term mentally ill: the MRC Needs for Care Assessment. *Psychological Medicine*, **17**, 971–981.

—— & —— (1993) The MRC Needs for Care Assessment: progress and controversies. *Psychological Medicine*, **23**, 837–841.

Cohen, J. A. (1960) A coefficient of agreement for nominal scales. *Educational and Psychological Measurement*, **20**, 37–46.

Department of Health Social Services Inspectorate (1991) *Care Management and Assessment: Summary of Practice Guidance*. London: HMSO.

Feinstein, A. R. & Cicchetti, D. V. (1990) High agreement but low kappa: I. The problems of two paradoxes. *Journal of Clinical Epidemiology*, **43**, 543–549.

Gardner, S. B., Winter, P. D. & Gardner, M. J. (1991) *CIA Confidence Interval Software*. London: British Medical Journal.

Grammatik Software (1992) *Grammatik 5 for Windows version 1.0*. Essex Reference Software International.

Hogg, L. I. & Marshall, M. (1992) Can we measure need in the homeless mentally ill? Using the MRC Needs for Care Assessment in hostels for the homeless. *Psychological Medicine*, **22**, 1027–1034.

Holloway, F. (1994) Need in community psychiatry: a consensus is required. *Psychiatric Bulletin*, **18**, 321–323.

House of Commons (1990) *The National Health Service and Community Care Act*. London: HMSO.

Maslow, A. H. (1954) *Motivation and Personality*. New York: Harper & Row.

Phelan, M., Wykes, T. & Goldman, H. (1994) Global function scales. *Social Psychiatry and Psychiatric Epidemiology*, **29**, 205–211.

Pryce, I. G., Griffiths, R. D., Gentry, R. M., et al (1993) How important is the assessment of social skills in current long-stay in-patients? *British Journal of Psychiatry*, **162**, 498–502.

Slade, M. (1994) Needs assessment: who needs to assess? *British Journal of Psychiatry*, **165**, 287–292.

——, Phelan, M., Thornicroft, G., et al (1996) The Camberwell Assessment of Need (CAN): comparison of assessments by staff and patients of the needs of the severely mentally ill. *Social Psychiatry and Psychiatric Epidemiology*, **31**, 109–113.

SPSS (1993) *SPSS for Windows version 6.0. Statistical Package for the Social Sciences*. Chicago: SPSS Inc.

Stevens, A. & Gabbay, J. (1991) Needs assessment needs assessment. *Health Trends*, **23**, 20–23.